LYME BRAIN

The impact of Lyme disease
on your brain and how
to reclaim your smarts!

BioMed Publishing Group, LLC

P.O. Box 550531

South Lake Tahoe, CA 96155

For our other Lyme disease books & DVDs, visit:

www.LymeBook.com

To purchase additional copies of this book, visit:

www.LymeBrainBook.com

978-0-9882437-7-4

DISCLAIMER

DEDICATION

This book is dedicated to every person
who is suffering from Lyme disease –
may you find healing and recovery,
and may you 'get your brain back.'

ACKNOWLEDGEMENTS

I want to thank my publisher Bryan Rosner for his ongoing support, his wise counsel, and the spirit of true partnership that he brings to our collaborations. Thank you also to my friend and editor Kim Junker – this is our fourth book together, and I feel like we're definitely on a roll!

I so appreciate the valuable time that was given by Bob Bransfield M.D., Leo Shea Ph.D., Sandy Berenbaum L.C.S.W., Scott Forsgren and Connie Strasheim – being able to share your words of wisdom was a great addition and will provide great information for our readers, so I am grateful for them giving their precious time to provide that. Thank you also Dr. Bransfield for writing the foreword – you have so much expertise in this area and it was so special to have your contribution. Steve Harris M.D., you mentored me during my early days of treating Lyme disease, and your support and endorsement mean a lot to me.

Thank you also to Michael and Dee Anne Canepa for having a last-minute read and putting their editing minds to work.

Thank you to my office staff, Brenda and Carmen, for taking so much off my shoulders so that I could carve out the time to write, and to Emily Poccia, N.D. for being willing to jump on a very steep learning curve to be able to care for many of our patients.

Finally, thank you to my ever-supportive husband Dave and my beautiful daughter Valentina. My family means everything to me and I couldn't do what I do without them providing a supportive and loving home base, and a strong foundation for me.

ALSO BY
NICOLA McFADZEAN DUCHARME, ND

※

*The Lyme Diet: Nutritional Strategies for Healing
from Lyme Disease*

*The Beginner's Guide to Lyme Disease:
Diagnosis and Treatment Made Simple*

*Lyme Disease in Australia:
Fundamentals of an Emerging Epidemic*

Purchase these and other Lyme disease books
by visiting www.LymeBook.com

TABLE OF CONTENTS

FOREWORD

by Robert C. Bransfield, M.D., D.L.F.A.P.A.

———◁◇▷———

Lyme Brain: The impact of Lyme disease
on your brain and how to reclaim your smarts!

I would like to thank Nicola McFadzean Ducharme, N.D. for taking on the effort to write *Lyme Brain: The impact of Lyme disease on your brain and how to reclaim your smarts!* More attention is needed on the mental symptoms associated with Lyme/tick-borne disease, and books addressing the mental symptoms are very much needed. Patients and family members need to be better informed on this subject.

Treating the mental symptoms seen with Lyme and associated diseases is both frustrating and rewarding. It is frustrating due to the complexity of these conditions and the obstacles that exist in the healthcare system, but it is also very rewarding when we can help patients navigate through multiple obstacles and improve from chronic debilitating symptoms. We were educated with very basic disease models that are insufficient when dealing with more complex diseases with multiple contributors, multiple pathophysiological processes and multiple symptom presentations. Multiple scientific disciplines need to be integrated to understand and effectively treat these conditions.

Microbes in our external and internal environment have a significant effect upon our health, and infections can have a significant impact upon our mental health even when they do not penetrate into the central nervous system. Psychiatric illness is always caused by something, and these causes need to be better understood. There are many who instead see psychiatric symptoms as a diagnosis by default when they cannot explain the cause of a symptom. Invariably, clinicians who follow this belief system lack sufficient training in tick-borne diseases, psychodynamics and neurophysiology, which explains an inability to understand the pathophysiology of mental symptoms. Our mental adaptive capabilities have been perfected by many years of evolution, and mental symptoms and mental illnesses do not spontaneously occur without a clear and significant cause. Although emotional trauma plays a contributing role in the etiology of some mental illness, a large number of mental illnesses are caused by physical injury to our nervous system from unknown and known causes, which often include infections and immune reactions to these infections. However, what causes a disease may not be the same as what causes that same disease to progress or persist, and these issues must be addressed as well. Implementing a multi-systems approach pulls together the components from multiple scientific disciplines that allow us to adapt to the complexity of these conditions.

When Polly Murray first drew attention to an epidemic of illness in Lyme, Connecticut, the physician investigating the outbreak was a rheumatologist. Since then, other rheumatologists, infectious disease specialists, bench scientists, microbiologists and others who lack psychiatric capability defined the disease from their limited perspectives and set policy and research planning decisions for the National Institute of Health and the Centers for Disease Control for Lyme disease that failed to incorporate psychiatric considerations. Other countries then follow the lead of these two institutions. To my knowledge, no psychiatrist knowledgeable about Lyme disease has ever been consulted when determining major policy decisions regarding Lyme disease at these institutions.

Although early symptoms are musculoskeletal, most of the later and more significant symptoms are psychiatric, cognitive and neurological. A few hundred articles in the peer-reviewed literature prove the association between neuropsychiatric symptoms and Lyme and other related tick-borne diseases. In spite of this, an influential group of policymakers are loyal to their belief systems based upon a 1970s definition of Lyme disease and discount the brain symptoms as being "subjective, non-specific and psychiatric." The blindness to comprehend the neuropsychiatric symptoms has stifled research, accurate epidemiology, medical education, patient awareness, treatment effectiveness and adequacy of insurance coverage. As a result, an epidemic of chronic mental illness associated with tick-borne diseases persists, is not being sufficiently addressed, and a large number of patients are feeling abandoned by our healthcare system.

We need humility when dealing with the complexities of Lyme disease. Borrelia has been found in ticks in amber in the Dominican Republic that were 15 to 20 million years old. This is an adversary with great adaptive capability. It has existed on this planet much longer than humans. Who has the greater chance of still being on this planet millions of years into the future—humans or *Borrelia*? When dealing with such a formidable adversary, patients need to consider multiple sources of information, do some of their own research, seek more than one opinion and be prepared to advocate for themselves. I hope this book helps to increase your creativity and your curiosity to learn more, and improves the quality of your life and health.

Robert C. Bransfield, M.D., D.L.F.A.P.A

INTRODUCTION

Lyme Brain. You all know exactly what I'm referring to. It's all the horrible brain manifestations of Lyme disease and its related infections. Many a Lyme patient has said to me, "Dr. Nicola, I can live with the pain, I can handle the fatigue, but I just can't cope with feeling so stupid. I used to be a smart person." Many would happily trade a kidney to "get their brain back." It's heartbreaking, because I see the impact that this has on the quality of life of so many people.

I know for a fact that you're not stupid, you're not losing your mind (although I get that it feels that way), and even if it seems to be lost, we can help you get it back again. I have seen patients with severe Lyme Brain experience remarkable recoveries. In fact, as I sit here writing, I'm thinking of a lady named Nikki, the previous president of the Lyme Disease Association of Australia (LDAA).[1] When she had active Lyme, she experienced terribly debilitating cognitive problems. She would get in the car, drive up the street and forget where she had set off to, so she would turn around and return home. She struggled to take care of her family. Today, she's working on her Ph.D., has successfully run the LDAA and definitely has her smarts back.

Lyme Brain also makes treatment harder, doesn't it? If it's not bad enough having to take a pile of pills and potions every day, Lyme Brain seems set out to sabotage your efforts. Keeping all those pills straight seems like a Herculean task, especially when Pill X can't be taken with Pill Y, and Potion B counteracts Potion A, and Herb 1 wants to be taken five minutes away from Herb 2, and Herb 3 yet another five minutes later. Medications and supplements run out before you realize you're out, and by then, figuring out how to get refills in time takes all your effort. Life is held together by pillboxes, reminder pings and alarms, and hopefully willing family members or friends who can help keep it all straight. It's hard to stick with the

---

[1] Cited with permission

3

treatment that can help get you better when your illness takes away your capacity to stick with the treatment that can help you get better. It's a vicious cycle.

Despite all of these challenges, recovery is possible, and you can get your brain back. You may never want to embark on a Ph.D. (I don't blame you!), but being able to go to the store and remember the five items you need without a shopping list, trusting yourself to pick up your children from sports practice, not having to worry about forgetting to turn off the stove, going back to a job you loved, and maintaining a healthy social life and personal relationships are all worthy aspirations that are attainable.

Lyme Brain isn't just about cognitive deficits, either. It often involves psychoemotional elements such as anxiety and depression. In fact, the majority of my patients experience anxiety and/or depression (usually both). Some people experience panic attacks while some get so anxious that they can no longer drive. Some people develop obsessive-compulsive tendencies or suicidal thoughts, nightmares and night terrors, and rage and impulsiveness. These, too, are tremendously hard to deal with.

Despite the number of Lyme patients who experience Lyme Brain—brain fog, short-term memory loss, difficulty with focus and concentration, anxiety, depression and the host of other aspects that make up the cognitive and neuropsychiatric aspects of Lyme—there is still limited information out there as to how to help the situation. This book aims to fill that void.

Section 1 explains what is actually occurring in the brain. It helps to understand some of the mechanisms of Lyme Brain because then it's easier to understand what to do to improve them. We'll discuss the role of inflammation and neurotoxins as well as the different co-infections of Lyme and how they impact the brain. We'll also outline some of the tools available to assess brain structure and function.

Sections 2 through 6 focus on solutions: the medications, supplements, therapies and modalities that can help Lyme Brain. Which antibiotics cross the blood-brain barrier? Do supplements for brain function really work? How can I adapt my nutrition to help my brain? How can I help my brain regenerate and heal even after the infections are dealt with? All these questions will be addressed. I also look at PTSD (post-traumatic stress disorder) in Lyme patients. PTSD is typically thought of as a syndrome that results from a major trauma such as a war or a horrific accident, but Lyme patients experience PTSD, too.

Section 7 discusses other barriers that may hinder recovery from Lyme disease, including heavy metals, mold and hormone imbalance.

Section 8 discusses Lyme Brain in children. Children may manifest neurological aspects of Lyme differently than adults, resulting in autism, PANDAS, bipolar disorder or learning difficulties. We'll take a look at the research and review some tools for helping children.

Section 9 guides you on how to put it all together and includes lists of my favorite products and protocols that can help with Lyme Brain.

Section 10 is a collection of interviews that I've done with both Lyme practitioners and patients. They share their stories, experiences and tips for helping you get well.

I hope that you find this book a valuable resource and that it propels you forward on your healing journey.

Yours in good health,

Dr. Nicola

San Diego, CA

ASSUMPTIONS OF THIS BOOK

In this book, Lyme disease refers not only to the textbook definition of infection with Borrelia burgdorferi, but also to the broader definition encompassing both Borrelia and its typical co-infections such as Babesia, Bartonella and Ehrlichia.

Lyme disease in this book also implies the many problems that accompany the infections, including hormone imbalance, toxicity, inflammation, emotional disturbances and nutritional deficiencies.

Therefore, most of the time when I use the term Lyme Brain, I am referring to the cognitive and neuropsychiatric aspects of all of these infections and disturbances. There will be sections that relate more to Borrelia itself, simply by virtue of the scientific studies and evidence presented, and in parts, I will attempt to speak specifically to the subtle nuances between the co-infections; however, there is so much overlap in symptomatology that it can be hard to separate.

> ## *Lyme Brain:*
> *brain fog, short-term memory loss, difficulty with focus and concentration, anxiety, depression and the host of other aspects that make up the cognitive and neuropsychiatric aspects of Lyme.*

SECTION 1:

FUNDAMENTALS OF LYME BRAIN

CHAPTER 1

THE SCOPE OF THE PROBLEM

In an article published in *Lyme Times*, 70% of Lyme disease patients report some extent of cognitive dysfunction.[1] In my opinion, that is a conservative estimate. Amongst my own patients, I see numbers closer to 90%.

Marian Rissenberg, Ph.D., and Susan Chambers, M.D. conducted a study of 49 Lyme patients who had been extensively evaluated using a complex battery of neuropsychological tests, a depression inventory and a symptom checklist.[2] Their findings showed that only 11% did not demonstrate any cognitive impairment, 63% demonstrated moderate cognitive impairment and 14% demonstrated severe cognitive impairment. It is interesting to note that *all* the patients evaluated reported cognitive issues, even the ones that did not test positive based on their evaluation and diagnostic criteria. In other words, the 11% that did not officially demonstrate cognitive impairment according to testing still thought they had it. It is also interesting that the patients with severe impairment actually met the diagnostic criteria for dementia, which shows just how destructive Lyme disease can be.

Their study also indicated that cognitive impairment in Lyme patients is less an issue of localized, focal damage in certain areas of the brain (as may be seen in a stroke victim, for example, where a specific area in the brain is damaged), but rather, the issues appear to be at the higher level integrative functions, more diffusely spread throughout the brain in complex neuronal systems. It's a more broadly spread issue, which can help us understand why its effects on cognitive and neurological function are so diverse.

The major types of cognitive challenges can be grouped into the following categories, as delineated by Rissenberg and Chambers:

❖ **Attention and mental tracking** – the ability to focus on one task to completion and the inability to multitask. This can lead to scenarios like the one where the Lyme patient drives down the street only to forget where she is going and has to turn around. During conversations, a Lyme patient may lose his or her train of thought or, if an interruption occurs, may be unable to return to the original train of thought or conversation.

❖ **Memory** – many Lyme patients report an issue with memory. According to the Rissenberg and Chambers study, the problem, in fact, is more about the difficulty processing and retrieving information rather than the storage of information itself. Nonetheless, the result for the Lyme patient feels the same. They have difficulty recalling information, forget where things are even within their own homes, forget appointments with doctors, and so on. This is what can make compliance with treatment regimens so difficult, and subsequently, patients need to adapt by making lists, setting alarms and reminders, and employing other tactics to help them remember.

❖ **Receptive language** – this involves understanding written and spoken language. For the Lyme patient, social interactions can be challenging, as they lose track of conversations and can't process what they're hearing quickly enough to comprehend it. Many Lyme patients report that they can no longer read due to the difficulty they face interpreting the words that they see on the page. One patient likened it to reading a foreign language—a slow and laborious process where one has to read the words, then do a translation in their head, try to register it in their native language and realize what those words mean, while at the same time starting the process with the next words in the line. It can be very time-consuming and exhausting.

❖ **Expressive language** – this is more about the ability to communicate using written and spoken words. The very common issue of word-finding difficulties falls under this category. Often I see this in consultations with my patients: they may have exerted a lot of effort to get to the appointment; they're often worried about having the incorrect time or being late; and they're stressed at having to function, be on time, speak for an hour and generally function in a way that will allow them to get the most out of the appointment. All this extra stress is challenging to start with, but then I see them struggling to explain how they're doing, communicate their challenges and find the language required to express themselves accurately. I see it take a real toll, and expressive language is one of the major areas hit.

A few years ago, I received a letter in an envelope addressed to me at my office. The writing looked like that of a child—it was shaky and barely legible. Inside were eight pages of writing—some of it was legible, but most of it was squiggles and circles in place of letters. I could decipher enough to know that this was from a Lyme sufferer, and it was an expression of her experience with her disease and a desperate cry for help, but I could see clearly that whether or not she was cognizant of what she was saying, there was a complete inability to communicate it using language. My heart broke for her, and although I will never know who sent it, I pray that she found help and a way out of her suffering.

❖ **Visuo-spatial processing** – these are more issues of spatial relations but are also linked to vision. Many Lyme patients cannot drive because their view of the world is distorted (and I mean that literally, not figuratively). They get lost, they lose objects easily and they don't have a sense of dimension and space. They can't tell how much space they have between them and the car in front or how wide they need to turn to navigate a corner successfully. Some of these issues can be linked to problems with the visual field and visual processing areas of the brain—that is, the areas related to eyes and eyesight—but typically it's a bigger issue than that. There's a spatial processing element to it, and this kind of processing happens deeper within the brain. Some of my patients describe it as being in a different dimension. Some say they lose depth perception altogether. Some feel like they're living in a movie where things seem very surreal, and some say it's like being on a really bad trip that won't end.

❖ **Abstract reasoning** – this is the ability to perceive issues and reach conclusions through generalizations rather than concrete factual information (i.e., one's ability and aptitude to reason logically and solve problems on a complex, intangible level—the ability to "get it"). It can involve the ability to think through ideas, decipher one concept from another, solve problems, and express creativity and judgment. Given that relationships between human beings rely on a lot of abstract reasoning, this can present great social and occupational problems for Lyme sufferers. For example, a person with compromised abstract reasoning may not be able to fully comprehend the impact of their actions. They may seem oblivious to certain repercussions of their actions on people around them simply because they cannot think through the more abstract elements of relationship. They may not be able to problem solve effectively in any relationship hiccups that occur. This can be very difficult for spouses, family members and friends of Lyme patients, who are trying their best to lend support but are sometimes gobsmacked (that's Australian for shocked) at some of their actions and what might seem like thoughtlessness. The Lyme sufferer, however, may be oblivious and simply can't see the consequences of their actions or decisions. Another example I see is when patients are presented with choices and options in their treatment protocols. While I treat my patients like fellow members of the medical team and recruit their input on treatment decisions, there are times when I have to recognize that they may be quite incapable of making decisions for themselves, and need to be told what to do and how to proceed.

❖ **Speed of mental and motor processing** – many Lyme patients report that they simply can't keep up with normal conversation speeds. Their brain can't hear, feed the information to the auditory processing center, interpret the information, think through a response and get it out of their mouths in a timely fashion. Their thought processes may be slower and their communication hindered. Again, I think of a person trying to keep up with a conversation that's in a foreign language in which they're not fluent; it's a real effort. I know that in my study of the French language, I'm so busy translating the first words in the sentence that by the time I have them figured out, I haven't heard the rest of the sentence, and I end up completely lost! I imagine this is exactly what it feels like for a Lyme patient, translating life as it's happening but constantly feeling left behind. Slower mental processing speeds also make it harder to meet deadlines, make appointments on time, and even cope with activities of daily living such as dressing and preparing food.

REFERENCES

[1] Rissenberg, M, and S Chambers. "Distinct pattern of cognitive impairment noted in study of Lyme patients." *Lyme Times* 20 (Jan-Mar 1998): 29-32.

[2] Rissenberg, M, and S Chambers. "Distinct pattern."

CHAPTER 2

DEPRESSION AND ANXIETY:
THE CHICKEN OR THE EGG?

———◇———

Depression and anxiety are among the more common symptoms reported by Lyme patients. Other mood-related issues include irritability, explosiveness, anger (aka "Lyme rage"), feelings of hopelessness, suicidal thoughts and obsessive-compulsiveness.

The question is, are such mood issues a result of the cognitive dysfunction or a separate issue altogether?

In Rissenberg and Chambers' study,[3] they concluded that the severity of cognitive impairment is so impactful and destructive to home, employment, marriage, social relationships and general wellbeing that the anxiety and depression are secondary to those factors.

Certainly the level of self-reported anxiety was highest in the group showing the most severe cognitive decline.

I do not disagree with them, but I believe there is more to it than that. I often tell my patients that anxiety and depression are a double-sided problem. Certainly, on one hand, anxiety and depression are a natural response to a debilitating chronic illness—an illness that can cause constant and horrific pain, render people housebound and bedbound, interfere with careers, relationships, social lives, marriages and the ability to participate in raising children, and essentially take away life as it was previously known. I think most people would feel pretty depressed given all of that. I know I would. Anxiety is also a natural response—how to pay for medical costs, how to keep the family functioning, how to choose the right doctor and treatment path, how to navigate the great unknown about levels of recovery and duration of treatment. These are termed reactive depression and anxiety and are considered adjustment disorders. In other words, the changes in mood are attributed to a stressful life event and will tend to resolve once the stressful event is removed. I see this in many of my patients. Their anxiety will naturally lift as they go through treatment and feel more positive and hopeful about the future.

The second cause of anxiety and depression is more organic. Lyme disease *creates* depression and anxiety, which are symptoms of the illness that are just as real as fatigue and joint pain. So while anxiety and depression can be seen within the context of natural responses to chronic illness and pain, they are also very real, stand-alone symptoms. Borrelia and its co-infections create anxiety and depression by interfering with parts of the brain responsible for regulating these feelings and by throwing mood-regulating chemicals off. Although anxiety and depression are symptoms of the illness, they are not who the person is. *You are not anxiety and depression. The Borrelia, its co-infections and associated imbalances are causing anxiety and depression within you.* Treat the infections and related problems adequately, and many times, the anxiety and depression will resolve.

I have found in many conversations with my patients that it is a relief to be told and continually reminded that they are not inherently anxious and depressed people; it is not who they are and who they will be forevermore. They are simply experiencing symptoms of their illness—caused by the bacteria—which will improve over time as their other symptoms improve.

REFERENCES

[1] Rissenberg, M, and S Chambers. "Distinct pattern of cognitive impairment noted in study of Lyme patients." *Lyme Times* 20 (Jan-Mar 1998): 29-32.

CHAPTER 3

WHAT ACTUALLY CAUSES LYME BRAIN?

⸺⸻✦⸻⸺

Before we discuss specific causes of Lyme Brain, let's get clear on two underlying premises. The first is that Lyme disease is a chronic infectious process, and that bacteria can and do persist in the body beyond the Infectious Diseases Society of America's "standard of care," which is a 14 to 21 day course of antibiotics. I'm not going to get into all the research supporting that general premise (for more detailed information, I refer you to my book *The Beginner's Guide to Lyme Disease*, which states the evidence clearly). The second premise is that the Borrelia spirochetes (and co-infections) can and do get into the brain itself. Therefore, a chronic infectious process can give rise to long-term exposure of brain tissue to spirochetes and other pathogens, which can have far-reaching consequences.

Evidence of spirochetes in the brain is not new. It is well established that the spirochetal bacteria that is behind syphilis, Treponema pallidum, causes progressive dementia and brain atrophy in the late stages of that disease.[1] Although Treponema and Borrelia are different pathogens, both are spirochetes, so we can draw some conclusions about the activity of one and how that might relate to the other. As one of my patients once said to me, "Dr. Nicola, Lyme disease is the new syphilis."

Some of the research that indicated that Borrelia spirochetes could get into the brain was done on Alzheimer's patients. Researcher Alan MacDonald was one of the first to find spirochetes in the brains of Alzheimer's patients on autopsy.[2] Examination confirmed that the spirochetes were Borrelia burgdorferi sensu stricto (one of the strains responsible for Lyme disease). In two cases, postmortem studies showed positive serology (on blood and cerebrospinal fluid) by Centers for Disease Control (CDC) standards. Neurofibrillary tangles were reactive with specific Borrelia burgdorferi (B. burgdorferi) antibodies, and Borrelia antigens were found.

In another study, spirochetes of various kinds were found in the brains of 14 Alzheimer's patients; they were not found in 13 controls. Three of these cases were identified as Borrelia burgdorferi sensu stricto.[3]

Yet another study detected Borrelia bacterial DNA by PCR in 5 of 16 Alzheimer's patients and only 1 of 16 controls.[4]

Judith Miklossy, M.D., Ph.D. conducted a review of all available data concerning spirochetes and Alzheimer's disease. The cumulative results showed that spirochetes of various kinds were found in the brains of more than 90% of Alzheimer's cases, and Borrelia burgdorferi was detected in 25.3% of cases.[5]

The correlation between Borrelia burgdorferi and Alzheimer's disease is intriguing. However, the purpose of presenting this research is to show that the Borrelia spirochetes can indeed penetrate the brain tissue. I also want to stress that there are many Alzheimer's patients who do not house Borrelia spirochetes in their brain, and not all Lyme patients are going to develop Alzheimer's disease. This is an important distinction to make. I don't want you all to read this and think that you're on the road to Alzheimer's disease – that is not the case at all. Yes, it's true that a subset of Lyme patients may develop Alzheimer's disease, but there are also other factors to consider such as genetic predisposition; perhaps they would have developed Alzheimer's disease even in the absence of Lyme disease.

Now that we have clearly established that Lyme disease infects the brain directly, let's look at the ways it can wreak havoc. We'll use the following points as a roadmap throughout the book to determine which treatments need to be used to stop these damaging processes.

DIRECT DAMAGE TO NERVE CELLS

We know that in the body, spirochetes can exist outside of cells or inside of cells. The intracellular invasion allows them some protection from host defenses, primarily our immune response.

Bacteria in the brain are invasive, too, and can invade neurons (nerve cells that conduct electrical impulses) and glial cells (supporting cells of the nervous system that do not conduct impulses).[6, 7] The invasion, and the following inflammatory cascade that results, can lead to death of the nerve cells.

Researchers back this up. *"The presence of B. burgdorferi DNA in tissue samples from areas with inflammatory changes indicates that direct invasion of B. burgdorferi may be the pathogenetic mechanism for focal encephalitis in LNB (Lyme Neuro-Borreliosis)."*[8]

Although this sounds dire—and not to make light of it, it can be—the neuronal death appears to be secondary to an inflammatory cascade triggered by the bacterial invasion. In other words, it appears to be the secondary inflammation rather than the pathogen itself that causes cell apoptosis.[9] There are ways to mediate such inflammation, which we'll discuss later. If we can mediate the inflammatory response, then we can minimize cell damage and cell death.

Borrelia may also cause demyelination of the white matter in the brain. The myelin sheath is a protective sheath that surrounds the axon of the nerve cell (the branch that juts out from the nerve cell and transmits the impulse). Myelin serves primarily to increase the speed of nerve transmission, getting the message from one cell to the next in the quickest, most efficient manner. There are several neurological diseases that involve demyelination, but the best known, perhaps, is multiple sclerosis (MS). Given that a subset of Lyme patients have been diagnosed with MS, it does raise the question of whether their primary diagnosis is truly Lyme disease but the diagnosis of MS was made based on similar findings on MRI studies. Unfortunately, there are no curative treatments for MS, and while Lyme treatment may not be quick or straightforward, I have seen Lyme patients who have also been diagnosed with MS improve with antibiotic treatment. This is often also evidenced by a reduction in white lesions on their brain MRI. So, determining whether MS is underlying Lyme disease can make all the difference in the world in a patient's prognosis.

There are several studies that demonstrate demyelination in Lyme patients. Many of the studies are case reports, so it is unclear exactly how prevalent this is, but as with anything in Lyme disease, my suspicion is that it most likely occurs more frequently than the literature would imply.[10]

One researcher, Vesna Briner, did make this statement:

> "The diagnosis of multiple sclerosis (MS), despite well-defined clinical criteria is not always simple. On many occasions it is difficult to differentiate MS from various non-MS idiopathic demyelinating disorders, specific and infectious inflammatory diseases or non-inflammatory demyelinating diseases. Clinicians should be aware of various clinical and MRI "red flags" that may point to the other diagnosis and demand further diagnostic evaluation. It is generally accepted that atypical clinical symptoms or atypical neuroimaging signs determine necessity for broad differential diagnostic work up. Of the infectious diseases that are most commonly mistaken for MS the clinician should take into account Whipple's disease, Lyme disease, Syphilis, HIV/AIDS, Brucellosis, HHV-6 infection, Hepatitis C, Mycoplasma and Creutzfeld-Jacob disease, among others."[11]

Another quote from a study out of Croatia:

> *"Demyelinating diseases of the central nervous system include a wide spectrum of different disorders that may resemble multiple sclerosis (MS). The diagnosis of MS is based on typical clinical and paraclinical criteria…If some of these criteria are atypical, diagnostic algorithm should be extended to some other procedures to exclude other diseases that can mimic MS not only in symptoms, signs or course of the disease but also in laboratory findings. In such a case, an alternative, better explanation for the clinical manifestations should be considered and performing specific tests is helpful to exclude alternative diagnoses."[12]*

Certainly there are enough references and articles stating that infectious processes can be a cause of demyelination and that differential diagnosis must include those things. I wonder, then, why some doctors are still so reluctant to consider chronic infections such as Borreliosis in a patient presenting with MS?

THE INFLAMMATORY RESPONSE

As mentioned above, direct impact of the pathogens on the nerve cells, which either causes demyelination or nerve cell death, is one way that Borrelia and its co-infections cause brain problems.

The second major mechanism is the inflammatory response. In fact, inflammation in the brain is perhaps the most significant cause of Lyme Brain.

Let's review some basic physiology. Inflammation can occur for a number of reasons, but notably in response to a pathogen in the body that the immune system is trying to fight. Even though it can seem like a bad thing, it's actually part of the body's protective response. Inflammation can involve not only white blood cells, but also blood vessels in the area and cells in the damaged tissue, too. It is only a bad thing when the immune system becomes *too* active or the inflammatory response is prolonged.

When there is a pathogen such as Borrelia, the immune system activates to counter the threat and kill the pathogen. In doing so, the white blood cells of the immune system go to the affected area.

A whole cascade of events follows, the details of which are beyond the scope of this book. Suffice it to say that there are a few key features that are part of the inflammatory process.

One of these features is the production of cytokines. Cytokines are small proteins that are released by various cells of the immune system and function to facilitate communication and signaling between various cells. They orchestrate the trafficking of immune cells, direct them to the sites of injury and influence immune cell function. They are released by a range of immune cells including B cells, T cells, macrophages and mast cells. In very simple terms, they are messengers and facilitators. Types of cytokines include chemokines, interleukins, interferons, lymphokines and tumor necrosis factors. Cytokines can also influence Th-1 and Th-2 balance within the immune system, which is significant in chronic infections such as Lyme disease.

Chronic Lyme patients are found to have high levels of cytokines such as interferon-gamma, IL-10, TNF-alpha, interleukin-6, interleukin-1b, interleukin-8, interleukin-12 and C-reactive protein. Some cytokines are anti-inflammatory (IL-10 for example); however, the majority of cytokines found in Lyme patients are pro-inflammatory.[13,14,15]

Chemokines are chemicals that induce the movement of cells towards an area of damage or inflammation. Many chemokines have been found in Lyme patients: chemokine ligands CXCL12, CXCL13, CCL2, CCL3, CCL4 and CCL5.[16,17]

Nitric oxide (NO) is another inflammatory mediator. Nitric oxide is a reactive molecule that can cause oxidative stress and cell damage, giving rise to further inflammatory processes. Higher levels of nitric oxide have been found in Lyme patients as opposed to healthy subjects. Nitric oxide also controls blood vessel dilation and constriction, so nitric oxide levels may play a role in the blood flow and oxygenation of cerebral vascular tissue in Lyme patients.[18,19]

One interesting characteristic of nitric oxide, however, is that it has been found to be toxic to the Lyme bacteria.[20,21]

In an article in the Townsend Letter (Feb/ Mar 2006),[22] Professor Robert W. Bradford and Henry W. Allen postulate that there might be a role for therapeutic agents that inhibit PDE-5, an enzyme that regulates c-GMP, which in turn influences nitric oxide. Medications that inhibit PDE-5 include sildenafil (Viagra), Cialis and Levitra. From a naturopathic standpoint, the amino acid arginine may have similar effects. Further research would be needed to determine whether this, indeed, is therapeutically significant and potentially beneficial for Lyme patients.

Another byproduct of immune activation is changes in the vascular system and blood clotting mechanisms. Inflammation creates increased dilation of the blood vessels and increased permeability in the vessel walls. This allows more fluid to move into the tissue space, giving rise to stasis of the blood cells in the vessels. This serves a worthwhile purpose: it allows white blood cells to move along the vessel walls to the site of injury (think of all the traffic on a freeway as it pulls over and stops on the side of the road to allow an ambulance through. If the traffic were flowing as it usually does, the ambulance would have a hard time making its way to the problem location). However, it can also lead to negative effects such as reduced oxygenation of the tissues.

So, we see that inflammation causes blood coagulation, but coagulation itself also has the capacity to regulate immune response, again, largely through the activation of various signaling molecules.[23]

Coagulation is balanced by the fibrinolytic system, which acts as an anticoagulant, preventing ongoing blood clotting. Anticoagulants also function to reduce cytokine production and protect the endothelial cells from the damage caused by inflammation.[24]

So you can see that while inflammation is a necessary part of immune response, it is not without its negative effects on the body.

Think of it like a military invasion. If an intruder comes onto home soil, the military (immune system) are going to counter that threat. They will first go to the location of the invasion, spreading out to the extent that the bad guys have spread out. They will come in with guns blazing and missiles firing. The goal is to kill as many of the baddies as possible with the least impact on the home turf, but in the process of the invasion, some collateral damage may occur. Yes, the military might kill at least some (hopefully all) of the bad guys, but they may also take out a few local civilians, buildings might get blown up, and infrastructures may be destroyed. Some of this may be necessary to contain the original threat, but it's certainly not the goal of the military's defense strategy. Hopefully, once the invaders are neutralized, rebuilding of home base can occur to repair any collateral damage.

And so it is with inflammation in Lyme disease. When the immune system tries to protect the body from an invasion by pathogens, baddies will be eradicated, but inflammation will occur as a byproduct, which can damage tissues and create symptoms of its own. This is one of the necessary secondary effects, but it is also the mechanism for much of the collateral damage that we see.

In chronic Lyme disease, collateral damage is often more extensive, due to the fact that the battle is ongoing over months and years, compared with shorter battles that occur in acute infections.

NEUROTOXINS

One of the ways that Borrelia burgdorferi may act to cause Lyme Brain is by releasing toxins in the brain and central nervous system. Neurotoxins are substances that enter nerve cells through the nerve endings, disrupting the function of the cell along the way. There are many sources of neurotoxins, both infectious and non-infectious in nature. Other examples are heavy metals, molds and Candida, as well as the chemicals that we are exposed to by the industrialized products and services we consume in modern society.

While the concept of a specific neurotoxin produced by Borrelia has been a controversial one, there is at least some research supporting it.

Researchers Cartwright, Martin and Donta presented an abstract at a conference in 1989, which identified DNA in the Borrelia bacterial genome that produces a neurotoxin. This was named BbTox1.[25]

This toxin is cited to be similar in structure to the botulinum toxin, belonging to a family of toxic proteins called zinc endoproteinases. Professors Bradford and Allen in their article in the Townsend Letter for Doctors and Patients (Feb/Mar 2006) claim that the Borrelia toxin works by disabling the neurotransmitter acetylcholine, which would then impact motor functions as well as psychoemotional states.

In reality, there is fairly limited research in this area. A PubMed search of *BbTox1* only revealed one match, a study from Poland citing the existence of BbTox1 but with no new information.[26]

Another possible mechanism of neurotoxicity secondary to Lyme disease may be increased levels of ammonia. David Jernigan, D.C., D.N.M., an integrative practitioner, founder of the Hansa Center for Optimal Health and developer of Jernigan Nutraceuticals, states that he discovered that the majority of Lyme patients have elevated levels of ammonia in their brain and potentially in other parts of their bodies, too, including the liver.

Here is an excerpt from Dr. Jernigan's blog:

> *"It would seem that Bb releases ammonia, which is converted to glutamine by way of the glutamine synthetase pathways, leading to localized swelling of astrocytes (brain cells). This ammonia-induced glutamine accumulation may cause dysfunction of astrocytes, which leads to impairment of vascular reactivity (other than through a decrease in arginine availability for nitrous oxide) and increased production of nitric oxide...It has been reported that many neurological problems are caused by either congenital or acquired hyper-ammonemia."*[27]

Dr. Dietrich Klinghardt, another well-known integrative doctor who works with many Lyme patients, also believes that ammonia in the brain may play a contributing role in Lyme Brain. He associates ammonia elevations with a condition called Kryptopyrroluria (KPU), also known as Hemopyrrollactamuria (HPU). This is a metabolic disorder that impacts one's ability to metabolize zinc, biotin, manganese, B6 and arachidonic acid.

Brain-related symptoms that may be associated with KPU include:

- Poor dream recall

- Nervousness/anxiety

- Pessimism

- Depression

- Paranoia/hallucinations

- Perpetual disorganization

- Mood swings/emotional lability

- Stress intolerance

- Poor short-term memory

- Substance abuse

- ADHD

- Autism

- Withdrawal

(List taken from reference below)

Dr. Klinghardt estimates the incidence of KPU in Lyme disease patients to be 80% or higher; in patients with heavy metal toxicity (lead, mercury, cadmium and others) over 75%; and in children with autism, over 80%.[28]

He states that as KPU is treated, high levels of ammonia tend to normalize.

Clearly, biotoxins and neurotoxins seem compelling and may well be a significant and under-acknowledged cause of Lyme Brain. Much more research is needed in this area. In the later sections, which address the treatment of Lyme Brain, we'll talk about the ways to minimize the effects of these neurotoxins.

NEUROTRANSMITTER IMBALANCE

Another contributing factor to Lyme Brain is neurotransmitter imbalance. This may be more of an effect than a cause; however, it is something that I frequently see in my patients and is prevalent enough to warrant a discussion here.

Neurotransmitters are brain chemicals that transmit impulses from one nerve cell to another. There are many different neurotransmitters and each has a different role and influence on brain function (so far, there are over 100 identified).[29] They play a central role in mood, cognition and emotional state.

Perhaps the best-known neurotransmitter is serotonin—so well known because many antidepressants function as selective serotonin reuptake inhibitors (SSRIs). They prevent serotonin from being discarded, and cause it to be recycled and reused in the brain. Why? Because low serotonin levels can cause depression (newer generation antidepressants work on a variety of pathways, but serotonin is still one of the more significant).

Some neurotransmitters are stimulatory, while others are inhibitory. By definition, this means that some are likely to promote a nerve impulse while others will inhibit it. In terms of how they affect people, some are more "awakening" and some are more "calming." Epinephrine and norepinephrine are examples of more stimulating neurotransmitters, while serotonin and GABA are more calming. Dopamine is related to emotional states, pleasure centers and motivation. Dopamine and norepinephrine together influence working memory. Acetylcholine relates to motor system function but also plays a role in emotion, learning and short-term memory.

Glutamate is the most prevalent excitatory neurotransmitter in the brain. While it is inherently an excitatory neurotransmitter, excessive glutamate can cause overstimulation in the brain and excitotoxicity. This has been implicated in a range of different neurological issues including ALS, epilepsy, autism and Parkinson's disease.

GABA is the most prevalent inhibitory neurotransmitter in the brain. GABA is often used clinically to treat anxiety and can be easily obtained in supplemental form. It has a very calming effect and a valuable role in Lyme treatment. GABA can also be used to balance excess glutamate.

Neurotransmitter imbalances will be discussed in more detail in the treatment section, as we can use amino acids to fuel certain pathways and help balance altered neurotransmitters. This can help stabilize mood as well as assist with focus, concentration and memory recall.

REFERENCES

[1] Noguchi, H, and J W Moore. "A demonstration of Treponema Pallidum in the brain in cases of general paralysis." *J Exp Med* 17, no. 2 (1913): 232-238.

[2] MacDonald, A B, and J B Miranda. "Concurrent neocortical borreliosis and Alzheimer's disease." *Hum Pathol* 18, no. 7 (Jul 1987): 759-761.

[3] Miklossy, J, et al. "Borrelia burgdorferi persists in the brain in chronic lyme neuroborreliosis and may be associated with Alzheimer disease." *J Alzheimers Dis* 6, no. 6 (Dec 2004): 673-681.

[4] Riviere, G R, K H Riviere, and K S Smith. "Molecular and immunological evidence of oral Treponema in the human brain and their association with Alzheimer's disease." *Oral Microbiol Immunol* 17, no. 2 (Apr 2002): 113-8.

[5] Miklossy, J. "Alzheimer's disease-a neurospirochetosis. Analysis of the evidence following Koch's and Hill's criteria." *J Neuroinflammation* 8 (Aug 2011): 90.

[6] Miklossy, J, S Kasas, A D Zurn, S McCall, S Yu, and P L McGeer. "Persisting atypical and cystic forms of Borrelia burgdorferi and local imflammation in Lyme neuroborreliosis." *J Neuroinflammation* 5, no. 4 (2008).

[7] Miklossy, J, et al. "Beta-amyloid deposition and Alzheimer's type changes induced by Borrelia spirochetes." *Neurobiol Aging* 27 (2006): 228-236.

[8] Oksi, J, et al. "Inflammatory brain changes in Lyme borreliosis. A report on three patients and review of literature." *Brain* 119 (Pt 6) (December 1996): 2143-54.

[9] Ramesh, G, L Santana-Gould, F M Inglis, J D England, and M T Philipp. "The Lyme disease spirochete Borrelia burgdorferi induces inflammation and apoptosis in cells from dorsal root ganglia." *J Neuroinflammation* 10 (July 2013): 88.

[10] Durovska, J, S Bazovska, J Pancak, M Zaborska, M Derdakova, and P Traubner. "Infection with B. burgdorferi s.l., and the CNS demyelinating disease. A case report." *Neuro Endocrinol Lett* 32, no. 4 (2011): 411-4.

[11] Brinar, V V, and M Habek. "Rare infections mimicking MS." *Clin Nuerol Neurosurg* 112 (2010): 625-628.

[12] Dezmalj-Grbelja, L, R Covic-Negovetic, and V Demarin. "Differential diagnosis and diagnostic algorithm of demyelinating diseases." *Acta Clin Croat* 48, no. 3 (2009): 345-8.

[13] Pohl-Koppe, A, K E Balashov, A C Steere, E L Logigan, and D A Hafler. "Identification of a T cell subset capable of both IFN-gamma and IL-10 secretion in patients with chronic Borrelia burgdorferi infection." *J Immunol* 160, no. 4 (February 1998): 1804-10.

[14] Soloski, M J, L A Crowder, L J Lahey, C A Wagner, W H Robinson, and J N Aucott. "Serum inflammatory mediators as markers of human Lyme disease activity." *PLos One* 9, no. 4 (April 2014): e93243.

[15] Bransfield, R C. "The psychoimmunology of lyme/tick-borne diseases and its association with neuropsychiatric symptoms." *Open Neurol J*, 2012: 88-93.

[16] Bransfield. "The psychoimmunology."

[17] Myers, T A, D Kaushal, and M T Phillip. "Microglia are mediators of Borrelia burgdorferi-induced apoptosis in SH-SY5Y neuronal cells." *PLos Pathog* 5, no. 11 (November 2009): e1000659.

[18] Ratajczak-Wrona, W, et al. "Nitric oxide in Lyme borreliosis. Evaluation of serum levels of nitric oxide and its biomarkers in patients with Lyme borreliosis." *Prog Health Sci* 3 (2013): 2.

[19] Garcia-Monco, J C, and J L Benach. "Mechanisms of injury in Lyme neuroborreliosis." *Semin Neurol* 17, no. 1 (March 1997): 57-62.

[20] Bourret, T J, J A Boylan, K A Lawrence, and F C Gherardini. "Nitrosative damage to free and zinc-bound cysteine thiols underlies nitric oxide toxicity in wild-type Borrelia burgdorferi." *Mol Microbiol* 81, no. 1 (July 2011): 249-73.

[21] Seiler, K P, Z Vavrin, E Eichwald, Jr., J B Hibbs, and J J Weis. "Nitric oxide production during murine Lyme disease: lack of involvement in host resistance or pathology." *Infect Immun* 63, no. 10 (October 1995): 3886-3895.

[22] Bradford, Robert W, and Henry W Allen. "Biochemistry of Lyme Disease: Borrelia Burgdorferi Spirochete/Cyst." *Townsend Letter, the Examiner of Alternative Medicine.* February/March 2006.

[23] Petägä, J. "Inflammation and coagulation. An overview." *Thromb Res* 127 , no. Suppl 2 (January 2011): S34-7.

[24] Esmon, C T. "The interactions between inflammation and coagulation." *Br J Haematol* 131, no. 4 (November 2005): 417-30.

[25] Cartwright, M J, S E Martin, and S T Donta. "More Evidence of Lyme Biotoxins: A Novel Toxin (Bb Tox 1) of Borrelia burgdorferi [Lyme disease]." *James Schaller, MD, MAR 50 Books & Top Journal Articles.* http://www.babesiabook.com/articles/morelymebiotoxinevidence.html (accessed 2015).

[26] Zajkowska, J M, and T Hermanowska-Szpakowicz. "New aspects of the pathogenesis of lyme disease." *Przegl Epidemiol* 56, no. Suppl 1 (2002): 57-67.

[27] Jernigan, D. "The Alkaline Brain: Lyme Borrelia-induced Hyper ammonemia." *Jernigan Neutraceuticals.* 2016. www.jnutra.com/Ammonia.html (accessed 2015).

[28] Forsgren, S. "Kryptopyrroluria (aka Hemopyrrollactamuria): A Major Piece of the Puzzle in Overcoming Chronic Lyme Disease." *Explore* 18, no. 6 (2009).

[29] "Neurotransmitter." *Wikipedia: The Free Encyclopedia.* March 1st, 2016. http://en.wikipedia.org/wiki/Neurotransmitter.

CHAPTER 4
CO-INFECTIONS AND THE BRAIN

We know that Babesia, Bartonella, Ehrlichia and other co-infections of Lyme can contribute greatly to Lyme Brain (accordingly, throughout the book, Lyme Brain includes the effects of these co-infections, too). Let's take a look at some of the specifics of the most common ones.

Babesia species are intracellular protozoan parasites—not bacteria—that live in the red blood cells. So while Babesia does not invade the nerve cells themselves in the same way that the Borrelia spirochetes do, they can still cross the blood-brain barrier and cause problems.

We sometimes talk about the blood-brain barrier as if it's a sheet of plastic housing around the brain, but in reality, the barrier itself is a network of capillaries within the brain. It is called the blood-brain *barrier* because it dictates what molecules can cross and which ones cannot, based on size, polarity and molecular structure. One of its major functions is to protect the brain from unwanted outsiders by disallowing their passage across the endothelial walls of the capillaries. Some substances can cross easily simply based on a concentration gradient, while others need protein carriers or energy pumps. This will come up again when we look at which antibiotics can cross the blood-brain barrier.

Keeping the bad guys out is as equally important as letting the good guys in. It is known that protozoa such as Babesia can cross the blood-brain barrier, even though all the exact mechanisms are not clear.[1] It is postulated, however, that the Babesia-infected red blood cells adhere to the vascular endothelium (the very thin layer of cells that line the capillaries). In doing so, they can cause sludging of the red blood cells in the capillaries of the brain, leading to higher levels of inflammation, and lower blood perfusion and oxygenation of the tissues.[2]

Bartonella, Ehrlichia and Rickettsia can also cross the blood-brain barrier and get into the brain. These are all bacteria and are common co-infections of Lyme.

As well as being one of the more common co-infections of Lyme, Bartonella is also a common problem because of its prevalence in cats. Dr. Mike Stone, a board certified internist at Tufts University, says, "Of the approximately 60 million pet cats in the United States, at least 20% are infected with Bartonella."[3]

There are many references to Bartonella encephalopathy in the literature as well as cited examples of positive PCR tests for Bartonella in brain tissue.[4,5] Infection of brain vascular cells is also documented.[6] With regard to Ehrlichia, some studies suggest that Ehrlichia chaffeensis may be more capable of penetrating the blood-brain barrier than Anaplasma phagocytophilum.[7]

When we talk about Lyme Brain, it can be very hard to sort out which infection/co-infection is creating which symptom. There is a lot of overlap. However, I can make some broad observations based on what I see in my patients, and this is backed up by the experience of other Lyme-literate physicians.

When I see the true cognitive deficits, such as the short-term memory loss, difficulty with focus and concentration, word-finding issues, difficulty forming words and slurring of speech, I generally consider that to be related to Borrelia itself. Anxiety and depression can be caused by Borrelia, too.

I typically see the co-infection Babesia cause brain symptoms such as a low to moderate generalized anxiety, feelings of impending doom, nightmares or night terrors, or vivid dreams.

In Bartonella, I tend to see more severe psychoemotional and neurological symptoms: seizures, panic attacks, suicidal thoughts, severe anxiety, obsessive-compulsive behaviors, severe mood swings, outbursts and antisocial behavior. One study noted that patients who had psychiatric symptoms relating to Bartonella required higher doses than others of benzodiazepines, antidepressants and antipsychotics in order to function normally.[8]

There is also evidence that Bartonella sufferers have higher rates of substance abuse. A study demonstrated that the number of Bartonella bacteria in alcoholic subjects was significantly higher than the controls. However, it is unclear whether Bartonella infections created psychiatric symptoms that might have predisposed an individual to use alcohol or drugs as coping mechanisms, or whether perhaps an alcoholic cohort may be immune-compromised and more susceptible to the bacteria. Perhaps both mechanisms are at play.[9]

As I said, these are broad generalizations. There will be many cases of overlapping symptoms and many cases where an individual may present co-infections differently than the above.

One of the ways to identify which co-infections are driving which symptoms is to follow their pattern throughout treatment. One of the reasons I believe that the actual brain fog, memory issues and difficulty with focus and concentration is Borrelia driven is because when I treat my patients with medications that primarily impact Borrelia and cross the blood-brain barrier, I see these symptoms improve, whereas the insomnia and wacky dreams tend to respond more to Babesia treatment. Really extreme psychiatric symptoms such as rages, and suicidal thoughts and behaviors, respond mostly to Bartonella treatment.

We must also consider "brain" symptoms in light of other symptoms. If a patient has pain on the soles of the feet, red striae (stretch marks) on their back and not a whole lot of joint pain but presents with low-grade anxiety and some brain fog, we must think Bartonella even though they are not manifesting the severe psychoemotional symptoms.

If someone else demonstrates really debilitating anxiety along with panic attacks, but they also have drenching night sweats and shortness of breath as key symptoms, we must put that in context and think of Babesia. As with any assessment and diagnosis in Lyme disease, we must consider lab work, history and complete symptom picture to get the clearest idea of what is impacting the patient the most.

REFERENCES

[1] Elsheikha, H M, and N A Khan. "Protozoa traversal of the blood-brain barrier to invade the central nervous system." *FEMS Microbiol Rev* 34, no. 4 (July 2010): 532-53.

[2] "Babesiosis." *Wikipedia: The Free Encyclopedia.* February 26, 2016. https://en.wikipedia.org/wiki/Babesiosis.

[3] Picard, Richard. "Bartonella: a Stealth Infection." *Dr. Richard Picard: Redefining Wellness.* March 29, 2015. http://www.nutritionalhealthnow.com/bartonella-a-stealth-infection/.

[4] Gerber, J E, J E Johnson, M A Scott, and K T Madhusudhan. "Fatal meningitis and encephalitis due to Bartonella henselae bacteria." *J Forensic Sci* 47, no. 3 (May 2002): 640-4.

[5] George, T I, G Manley, J E Koehler, V S Hung, M McDermott, and A Bollen. "Detection of Bartonella henselae by polymerase chain reaction in brain tissue of an immunocompromised patient with mutliple enhancing lesions. Case report and review of the literature." *J Neurosurg* 89, no. 4 (1998): 640-4.

[6] Varanat, M, R G Maggi, K E Linder, and E B Breitschwerdt. "Infection of human brain vascular pericytes (HBPVs) by Bartonella henselae." *Med Microbiol Immunol* 202, no. 2 (April 2013): 143-51.

[7] Park, J, K S Choi, D J Grab, and J S Dumler. "Divergent interactions of Ehrlichia chaffeensis-and Anaplasma phagocytophilum-infected leukocytes with endothelial cell barriers." *Infect Immun* 71, no. 12 (December 2003): 6728-33.

[8] Schaller, J L, G A Burkland, and P J Langhoff. "Do Bartonella Infections Cause Agitation, Panic Disorder, and Treatment-Resistant Depression?" *MedGenMed* 9, no. 3 (2007): 54.

[9] Rolain, J M, D Arnoux, D Parzy, J Sampol, and D Raoult. "Experimental infection of human erythrocytes from alcoholic patients with Bartonella quintana." *Ann N Y Acad Sci* 990 (June 2003): 605-11.

CHAPTER 5

IS DAMAGE TEMPORARY OR PERMANENT?

This is the question on everyone's mind. Of course, when you're experiencing memory loss, you can't focus well enough to continue working at your job. You can't read a full page of a book without having to take breaks, and your mind generally doesn't function well enough to carry out what you need to do in your life. The terrifying part is not knowing whether it's going to last forever or if, indeed, there is hope of recovery. That is very natural and understandable.

I have some bad news, but I have much good news as well.

Yes, there are some cases where there appears to be permanent damage. When the brain has been under toxic and infectious assault for many years unchecked, there may be some permanent damage. Some people find that they never get back to the full capacity of their mind as they knew it previously or there may be a residual psychoemotional impact. This may be due to the effects of long-term inflammation such as tissue damage, hypoperfusion (low blood supply) leading to low oxygenation and tissue injury, impacts of toxic insults (including such things as heavy metals) and residual infections such as Candida and viruses that may impact the brain even beyond Lyme treatment. It is hard to say to what extent ongoing brain symptoms are due to actual irreversible damage, versus the chronicity of Lyme infection itself, or ongoing cofactors such as Candida, mold and other toxins.

But let's move on to the good news. I find that the majority of people with Lyme Brain can find resolution or, at the very least, significant improvement of their symptoms. Remember Nikki from the introduction—from forgetting where she was driving to, to writing her Ph.D. dissertation? That's quite the recovery, and I see those kinds of recoveries frequently.

If we go back to the root causes of Lyme Brain—infection, inflammation, neuro-toxins and neurotransmitters—each of those things can be addressed. I will expand more in the next section, but in broad terms, there are antimicrobials that cross the blood-brain barrier to kill off the pathogens in the brain; there are treatments that reduce the inflammatory response and dietary principles that help, too; there are detox therapies to help rid the body of toxins; and there are various ways to support neurotransmitters to help balance those out. I'm not saying it's quick or easy, but I have seen remarkable improvements and recoveries in people who started out very, very ill with horrible Lyme Brain and are now back at work, running their families and living their lives as productive, happy people.

There are also some old assumptions about the loss of neurons in the brain that are being debunked by scientific research right now, and that's even more good news.

We discussed earlier that Lyme could cause neuronal cell death. Historically, it was believed that neurons (cells in the nervous system) once dead could not regenerate, that we are born with a certain number of neurons and once they are gone, that's it, they're gone forever. That would be bad news for a Lyme patient with neurological Lyme, as cell damage from the infectious process would be unrecoverable.

Excitingly, there are two significant findings now that are challenging that old theory. The first is that adults can grow new neurons. Researchers at Princeton University have found that new neurons are constantly being added to monkeys' brains—mostly in the cerebral cortex, which is the largest and most advanced part of the brain. Within the cerebral cortex, the researchers found neurogenesis in three areas: 1) the prefrontal region, which controls executive decision making and short-term memory; 2) the inferior temporal region, which plays a crucial role in the visual recognition of objects and faces; and 3) the posterior parietal region, which is important for the representation of objects in space.[1] Much research still needs to be done, but this might provide incredible opportunities for therapy in degenerative diseases, such as Alzheimer's, as well as neurological infectious illnesses such as Lyme disease. Just knowing that the brain has that capacity and that it could be happening in your brain right now is encouraging!

The second is the area of neuroplasticity. I won't go into too much detail here because I will discuss it more later. Basically, neuroplasticity is the concept that the brain is changeable and malleable, and can respond to changes in behavior, external stimuli, environment and injury if need be. It is a fascinating area of study, and if you are interested in it, I highly recommend the book *The Brain That Changes Itself*.[2] There is evidence that if certain parts of the brain are damaged, other areas of the brain can take over the function previously performed by the injured part of the brain. This is especially important in situations such as strokes, where a focal, specific area of the brain is damaged, but is also relevant for Lyme patients where damage tends to be more diffuse.

I also think that neuroplasticity has major application for one's mental outlook and attitude towards their illness. The more a person chooses a certain thought or thought pattern, the stronger the neurological pathways for that thought pattern become. Therefore, if a person continually chooses thoughts of healing and recovery, they are actually supporting their brain in creating healing and recovery, and weakening the thoughts that are negative and hopeless. More on this later, but to me, this is a very profound concept and could make a world of difference in one's recovery from Lyme Brain.

Finally, there are also certain agents—herbs, supplements, etc.—that can help relieve Lyme Brain symptoms while the underlying causes are being addressed. Obviously, dealing with the root cause—the infection—is going to bring the lasting recovery that patients desire, but there's nothing wrong with helping with some of the symptoms and giving the brain a little boost while that process is taking place. These will also be discussed in Section 3.

REFERENCES

[1] Gould, E, A J Reeves, M S Graziano, and C G Gross. "Neurogenesis in the Neocortex of Adult Primates." *Science* 286 (October 1999).

[2] Doidge, N. *The Brain That Changes Itself: Stories of Personal Triumph from the Frontiers of Brain Science.* New York: Penguin Books, 2007.

CHAPTER 6

ASSESSING THE PROBLEM:

TESTS AND STUDIES

―――※○※―――

There are various tools that your doctor might employ to help assess what is causing your Lyme Brain. Well, let me rephrase that. We know that infection and inflammation are causing your Lyme Brain, but there are some tests that can help evaluate the degree and type of damage, and this can provide insight into how to improve the situation. Assessments can also help rule out other issues that could be contributing to the problem and co-existing alongside the Lyme disease.

In broad terms, we can classify these tests as either assessing the *structure* of the brain or assessing the *function* of the brain.

MRI
One of the main tools that doctors use to evaluate the neurological elements of Lyme is magnetic resonance imaging (MRI), which is a *structural* evaluation of the brain. It is used to assess areas of demyelination, but it can also measure inflammatory changes in the brain. Both of these are represented by white matter hyperintensities, or white lesions in the brain. Many of my patients who have had an MRI showing white matter are terrified that they have multiple sclerosis, but this is not necessarily true. Yes, one of the diagnostic criteria of MS is white lesions on the brain as seen on MRI, but that does not mean that white lesions automatically mean MS. In fact, many people without any major health issues would show white lesions that arise naturally with age.

It is thought that approximately 40% of Lyme patients have hyperintensities in the brain.[1]

Some studies demonstrate even higher percentages. The table below gives some examples.

Author	No. pts studied	No. w/pos findings	%
Fernandez[2]	14	6	43
Kruger[3]	3	3	100
Agosta[4]	20	12	60
Aalto[5]	16	12	75

While white matter lesions are the most common finding on MRIs, there may also be cranial nerve root or meningeal enhancements (the meninges are the protective membranes that surround the brain and line the skull). One study suggested that these findings are more common than is widely accepted and may provide useful assessment information for Lyme patients.[6]

White lesions in the brain can improve, and indeed resolve, with appropriate antimicrobial therapy. This is another way to differentiate positive MRI-findings in Lyme disease versus MS (which would not necessarily be responsive to antimicrobial therapy). However, it may take many months for the lesions to resolve, as the brain takes time to heal even following successful antibiotic treatment.

A newer technology called NeuroQuant is now being used to assess brain changes in Lyme patients (and other neurodegenerative conditions). This software is capable of measuring brain atrophy (shrinkage) in the hippocampus and other brain structures. It may detect neurological changes earlier, which allows for an earlier intervention. This is certainly also the goal in patients with dementia and Alzheimer's disease. This technology may also provide a better reflection of treatment response.

This is a relatively new technology, and its usefulness in Lyme disease is yet to be seen. However, in a field where accurate diagnostic information is quite hard to come by, it does have the potential to help assess the extent of neurological involvement and damage. Some doctors also use NeuroQuant MRI to decipher between the impacts of Lyme disease versus mycotoxins on the brain. As these things present very similarly from a clinical standpoint, this could be one of the most useful applications of it.

CT Scans

Computerized tomography (CT) scans are another assessment tool for structural elements of the brain. They are used with Lyme patients far less frequently than the MRI but are sometimes performed to rule out other issues such as tumors. CT scans are not considered to be adequate assessments for neuro-Borreliosis, and so they are not generally recommended. Many Lyme patients have had CT scans along the long road of their illness and their quest for a clear diagnosis, but in a person with known Lyme trying to get clear reflective information about the impact of their illness, the MRI is the preferred method of structural imaging.

SPECT Scans

While MRI and CT scans assess the *structure* of the brain tissue, SPECT scans can help to assess *function*. SPECT stands for Single Photon Emission Computer Tomography. It is somewhat controversial, however, and not all members of the medical community support it. They claim that it is unsuitable for diagnostic purposes and doesn't really help guide treatment protocols. In many cases, it does not receive insurance coverage, whereas an MRI is more likely to. Therefore, one of the criticisms of SPECT is the out-of-pocket costs to the patient relative to the usefulness of the diagnostic information. Another one of its limitations is that it cannot differentiate the possible cause of the findings. Lupus, HIV, chronic cocaine use or vasculitic inflammatory disorders may cause similar findings as Lyme disease.

Having said that, the SPECT scan can provide information that MRI and CT scans cannot and may still provide some objective measure of abnormalities in a disease in which it can be hard to produce solid objective findings. Indeed, It can provide evidence of a physiological basis of cognitive or psychoemotional symptoms, as opposed to those symptoms having a psychiatric cause.

One of the key findings on a SPECT scan is hypoperfusion, meaning diminished blood flow to certain areas of the brain. The most common finding is heterogeneous diffuse hypoperfusion. This may indicate vasoconstriction, which could then be mediated by vasodilating medications and/or supplements. SPECT may also be helpful in assessing the success of treatment regimens; improvement in perfusion of the brain may result from successful antimicrobial therapy.

One study of 183 people who met the clinical definition of chronic Lyme disease showed that a full 75% of them demonstrated abnormalities in blood perfusion to the brain. In the same patient cohort, 14% showed abnormalities on their MRIs. Treatment with antibiotics led to the improvement or resolution in symptoms over a 1–2 year period.[7] Therefore, even when an MRI appears normal, the SPECT scan can give useful evidence of problems in the brain.

The PET Scan

The Positron Emission Tomography (PET) scan is another functional assessment that extends beyond regional blood flow to also show regional brain tissue metabolism. Because it is much more expensive and more difficult to access than the

SPECT, it is not utilized extensively in clinical settings. The PET scan is also some-what more precise and specific than the SPECT scan, and for these two reasons, it is utilized more extensively in research settings.

The premise of the SPECT and the PET scans is that there is a relationship among brain glucose metabolism, brain blood flow and brain nerve activity. For this rea-son, gathering as much information as possible on these variables can be benefi-cial. Changes in both blood flow and metabolism can help explain problems with nerve function and, hence, neurological symptoms.

PET studies can also demonstrate continued brain effects even after the "standard of care" period of antibiotics. A study done by the Columbia University Lyme and Tick-Borne Diseases Research Center assessed whether changes in blood flow and regional brain metabolism continued in chronic Lyme disease beyond the initial antibiotic treatment. Using PET imaging as their assessment tool, they studied 35 patients and 17 healthy control subjects. Patients had prior, well-documented Lyme disease, a currently reactive Western Blot, prior treatment with at least three weeks of intravenous cephalosporin and objective memory impairment. They found that patients had ongoing abnormalities in functional brain activity, both in terms of per-fusion and metabolism.[81] This shows that the Infectious Diseases Society of America position on the efficacy of three weeks of IV antibiotics is clearly incorrect as it re-lates to regaining healthy brain function (amongst many other things!).

Recent reports from Dr. James Moeller of the Columbia Lyme Center suggest that there is a specific neural circuit that may be associated with the production of antibodies in the central nervous system and can be measured using a PET scan. This specific finding requires a PET scan and not a SPECT scan. If further research proves that this is clinically relevant and highly valuable, then PET scans might be more clinically applicable. In the meantime, the reality of cost and availability make SPECT scans a more accessible choice.

Neurotransmitter Tests

We have already discussed how neurotransmitter imbalances, which can poten-tially cause anxiety and depression, and contribute to cognitive issues such as sluggish thinking, memory loss and lack of focus/concentration, are a key feature in Lyme Brain.

Neurotransmitter levels in the body can be measured using both blood and urine samples. I typically utilize the urinary testing, as the sample can easily be collected by the patient at home and sent directly to the lab for analysis.

Urinary testing for neurotransmitters measures many of the primary neurotrans-mitters: serotonin, epinephrine, norepinephrine, GABA, glycine, histamine and glutamate. Some panels also include metabolites of neurotransmitters, such as 5-HIAA and DOPAC, to help with the assessment of serotonin and dopamine, respectively. By looking at the metabolites as well, we can see where blockages or bottle necks in the pathways may be occurring, which can help guide how to supplement specific amino acids to get things flowing more freely.

Blood tests for neurotransmitters do exist; however, serum testing is not suggested for assessments of neurotransmitters relating to Lyme Brain because of the low levels of neurotransmitters in the serum. This method of testing is better for evaluating dramatic changes in levels due to tumors and so on.

Platelet testing is considered somewhat more accurate than urinary testing; however, it can also be more difficult to access. Vitamin Diagnostics Lab in New Jersey is one of the few labs that offer it. That same lab conducted a study in 2005 to see which tests for neurotransmitters seemed to match the CSF levels the best (CSF is known to be the most accurate, but testing it is not practical in clinical settings). They found that platelet testing was the closest to CSF, followed by urine testing and then serum testing.[9]

Despite this finding, I do find urinary neurotransmitter testing to be helpful in evaluating neurotransmitter levels, and this can be helpful in guiding therapy with either antidepressant medication or amino acid therapy.

Neuropsychiatric Testing

Self-reports and questionnaires can be simple and inexpensive tools for practitioners to gather information and for patients to document their experiences with Lyme Brain, but bear in mind that this is subjective information and, therefore, may not be highly accurate. A person with Lyme Brain might not have the best memory of their own functionality or an accurate perception of issues such as mood swings, depression and anxiety levels. It is the role of the practitioner to ask comprehensive questions to gather as much useful information as possible as to the person's level of functioning. For patients, it is so important to be brutally honest with your doctor or practitioner, even though there may be feelings of embarrassment or shame in sharing your story. If you are having hallucinations or suicidal thoughts, or are just embarrassed that you didn't remember your daughter's name yesterday, practitioners are not there to judge but to help you through it and guide you towards recovery. The more information we have, the better we can help you.

Dr. Robert Bransfield has developed a great example of a neuropsychiatric questionnaire and he has kindly shared that with us (see Appendix B). Most Lyme-literate practitioners will have a subjective questionnaire to gather similar information, but Dr. Bransfield, as a Lyme-literate psychiatrist, has certainly created a comprehensive version that may be helpful for patients and other practitioners alike. Sandy Berenbaum, L.C.S.W. has also shared her assessment tool, which is highly succinct and easy to adopt (see Appendix A).

There are also more formal neuropsychiatric testing tools that do gather objective information and data as to a person's cognitive function. These are standardized tests and cover a wide array of traits, from verbal and visual memory to verbal fluency, concentration and attention, processing speed and executive functioning.

Examples of neuropsychiatric tests include the California Verbal Learning Test, the Controlled Oral Word Association Tests, an array of timed tests for processing speed, the Weschler Adult Intelligence Scale and the Word Memory Test.

It is also suggested for Lyme patients to include assessments of emotional status, such as the Beck Depression Inventory, the Beck Anxiety Inventory, the Depression Anxiety Stress Scale 42 and the Differential Assessment of Post-Traumatic Stress Inventory.

The typical Lyme-literate medical doctor is not likely to be equipped to offer this level of neuropsychiatric testing; this is more the domain of the Lyme-literate psychiatrist or psychologist. (The Columbia Lyme Center offers a very comprehensive battery of neuropsychiatric testing.) However, all Lyme-literate practitioners should include some assessment of psychoemotional and cognitive status in their patient intakes and interviews.

REFERENCES

[1] "Spinal Fluid and Brain Tests." *Lyme and Tick-Borne Diseaes Research Center.* http://www.columbia-lyme.org/patients/ld_spinal_fluid.html.

[2] Fernandez, R E, M Rothberg, G Ferencz, and D Wujack. "Lyme Disease of the CNS: MR imaging findings in 14 cases." *AJNR Am J Neuroradiol* 11, no. 3 (1990): 479-481.

[3] Kruger, H, E Heim, B Schuknecht, and S Scholz. "Acute and chronic neuroborreliosis with and without CNS involvement: a clinical, MRI, and HLA study of 27 cases." *J Neurol* 238, no. 5 (1991): 271-280.

[4] Agosta, F, M A Rocca, B Benedetti, R Capra, C Cordioli, and M Filippi. "MR imaging assessment of brain and cervical cord damage in patients with neuroborreliosis." *AJNR Am J Neuroradiol* 27, no. 4 (2006): 892-894.

[5] Aalto, A, J Sjowall, L Davidsson, P Forsberg, and O Smedby. "Brain magnetic resonance imaging does not contribute to the diagnosis of chronic neuroborreliosis." *Acta Radiol* 48, no. 7 (2007): 755-762.

[6] Agarwal, R, and G Sze. "Neuro-lyme disease: MR imaging findings." *Radiology* 253, no. 1 (October 2009): 167-73.

[7] Donta, S T, R B Noto, and J A Vento. "SPECT brain imaging in chronic Lyme disease." *Clin Nucl Med*, no. 37 (September 2012): e219-22.

[8] Fallon, B A, et al. "Regional cerebral blood flow and metabolic rate in persistent Lyme encephalopathy." *Arch Gen Psychiatry* 66, no. 5 (May 2009): 554-63.

[9] Audhya, T. "Advances in measurement of platelet catecholamines at Sub-picomole level for diagnosis of depression and anxiety." *Clinical Chemistry* 151, no. 6 Supplement (2005).

SECTION 2:

PHARMACEUTICAL APPROACHES TO LYME BRAIN

CHAPTER 7

INTRODUCTION

⸺⧓⸺

We've seen that Lyme Brain has several different causes and components. In this section, we are going to discuss the various medications that can potentially address Lyme Brain, including antibiotics, mood-regulating medications, medications for cognition and so on.

Clearly, treatments need to address the cause to affect lasting change. Some treatments are palliative, which means that they help reduce symptoms or provide relief. Sometimes palliative treatments and modalities get criticized for just putting a "Band-Aid" over the problem and "not getting to the root cause of the issue." My personal view is that there is nothing wrong with providing relief *while working on the underlying cause*. Palliative care is only a problem if it is the only care provided and is used to the exclusion of anything else—that is, done without any concurrent treatment to address the underlying problem.

Okay, with that established, let's get started. For the sake of organizing information, I am going to discuss medications in this section, then move on to natural treatments and nutrition in the remaining sections. This does not necessarily imply that I think medications are always superior or that they always work better, but I realize that if you have Lyme Brain, it might help to map out the information as clearly as possible!

CHAPTER 8

ANTIOBIOTIC THERAPY

———⊰⊱———

So what is the bottom line? In order to affect lasting change in Lyme Brain, we must minimize or eradicate the infection in the brain. One of the primary tools we have to do that is antibiotics.

To make a lasting difference, antibiotics must be able to cross the blood-brain barrier. Not all antibiotics cross the blood-brain barrier and address infection in the brain, and in fact, many of the medications used in Lyme treatment do not either. Hence, they can help other systemic symptoms and reduce total microbial load overall, but they just won't have the impact on neurological and Lyme Brain-related symptoms that others might. To be effective for Lyme Brain, your protocol must include antibiotics that cross the blood-brain barrier.

WHAT IS THE BLOOD-BRAIN BARRIER?
Let's review.

It's tempting to think of the blood-brain barrier as a solid covering that houses the brain, a layer of membrane or solid connective tissue that we can see as a definite entity, like a bag that the brain is carried around in, but this is not the case. The blood-brain barrier is actually composed of tight junctions between the cells lining the capillary walls. The "barrier" is more a correlate of the cells of tiny blood vessels and, in particular, the lipid membranes of those capillaries.

This design allows certain things to cross while keeping others out. For example, glucose and amino acids are substances that must be able to cross. Glucose is the brain's primary fuel source, and without it, we'd all be in trouble. Amino acids are the building blocks that make up protein and also cross easily.

Some substances diffuse across the barrier simply on a concentration gradient; that is, the molecules will move from an area of high concentration to low concentration without requiring any other input or fuel to do so. Some substances move across membranes using active transport mechanisms, such as pump systems, that move things in and out of cells, which can require energy. These different mechanisms can be significant for drug transport across the blood-brain barrier. For example, giving antibiotics intravenously will increase the concentration of it, which can facilitate greater movement across the lipid membranes of the capillaries.

WHAT DETERMINES WHICH ANTIBIOTICS CROSS THE BLOOD-BRAIN BARRIER?

There are certain features that allow greater movement of antibiotics across the blood-brain barrier. Each medication has a combination of the following properties, and this combination dictates how easily it penetrates the blood-brain barrier.

MOLECULAR SIZE

The size of each molecule of any given antibiotic will greatly influence its ability to cross into the central nervous system; the smaller the molecular mass, the more likely it is to penetrate.

LIPOPHILICITY

Lipophilicity refers to the extent to which the molecule is attracted to fatty molecules so that they can attach to, and pass through, lipid cell membranes. Given that lipid membranes surround all cells and that there is at least one cell layer surrounding the entire brain, there are at least two lipid membranes that all substances must pass through. If the medications are molecules that repel fatty acids, they will resist those membranes and, therefore, have a compromised ability to pass through. Fat-loving antibiotic molecules will be drawn to those lipid membranes and, consequently, are more able to pass through.

PLASMA PROTEIN BINDING

The ability to bind to plasma proteins is another determinant of a medication's ability to pass through into the central nervous system. The more a molecule is bound to proteins, the less free it is to cross the blood-brain barrier.

There is one condition in which all of the above go out the window. If there is extreme inflammation, such as in meningitis, the blood-brain barrier becomes "leaky." In severe inflammation, the list of antibiotics that can be used expands, because with the extent of inflammation, the junctions open up and larger antibiotic molecules can pass through.

Even though there is inflammation in Lyme disease, it is not as acute and profound as in meningitis. It can be confusing to see a medication, such as cefdinir, utilized for meningitis treatment when it is not generally considered a great medication for CNS penetration. The severity of the inflammation is the determining factor.

A REVIEW OF THE ANTIBIOTICS USED IN LYME TREATMENT

To help put this in perspective, let's do a quick recap of the different categories of antibiotics often used in Lyme treatment.

The Borrelia bacteria can exist in three different forms: spirochete, cell-wall deficient and cyst form. Different antibiotics address different forms due to the way they work. For example, an antibiotic that works by shooting holes in the bacterial cell wall (so to speak) might be good for the spirochete forms but will not be good for the cell-wall deficient forms, which as the name suggests, do not have a formed cell wall in which to shoot holes. Hence, we end up needing one medication from each category to thoroughly address Borrelia.

Here are the categories with some examples of the medications used. This list is by no means exhaustive but represents some of the more common medications prescribed.

COMMONLY USED MEDICATIONS FOR BORRELIA

SPIROCHETE FORMS

Cephalosporin family

        Examples: Ceftriaxone (Rocephin)
                                    Cefuroxime (Ceftin, Zinnat)
                                    Cefdinir (Omnicef)

Penicillin family

        Examples: Amoxicillin (Amoxil)
                                    Penicillin G Benzathine (Bicillin L-A)

CELL-WALL DEFICIENT FORMS

Tetracycline family

        Examples: Doxycycline (Doryx, Vibramycin)
                                    Minocycline (Minocin, Dynacin)

Macrolides

        Examples: Azithromycin (Zithromax)
                                    Clarithromycin (Biaxin, Klacid)

CYST FORMS

Examples: Tinidazole (Tindamax, Simplotan, Fasigyn)
Metronidazole (Flagyl)
Hydroxychloroquine (Plaquenil)

COMMONLY USED MEDICATIONS FOR CO-INFECTIONS

BABESIA

Examples:

Atovaquone (Mepron)
Atovaquone/ Proguanil (Malarone)
Artemether/ Lumefantrine (Riamet, Coartem)
Nitazoxonide (Alinia)

BARTONELLA

Examples:

Rifampin (Rifadin, Rifampicin)
Levofloxacin (Levaquin)
Ciprofloxacin (Cipro)

EHRLICHIA

Examples:

Doxycycline (Doryx, Vibramycin)
Minocycline (Minocin, Dynacin)

Now that you have that framework to reference, you can see where the following medications fit into the treatment protocol. Let's now look at some of the optimal antibiotics for crossing the blood-brain barrier.

ANTIBIOTICS THAT CROSS THE BLOOD-BRAIN BARRIER
CEFTRIAXONE

The cephalosporin family of antibiotics is used to treat spirochete forms of Borrelia. In general, as a family, they are not known to have great penetration of the blood-brain barrier. However, despite mixed research on blood-brain barrier penetration, one medication in that family stands out clinically as a stellar medication for neurological Lyme.

Ceftriaxone, often known by its brand name Rocephin, is one of the best-known Lyme medications and is certainly the preeminent one given intravenously (via IV).

It is a third generation cephalosporin and works by weakening and then causing the demise of the bacterial cell wall.

It does cross the blood-brain barrier, especially since it is given intravenously and, hence, high enough doses can be given to reach therapeutic concentrations. Ceftriaxone can be given intramuscularly also, but that is neither practical nor as effective in Lyme treatment.

Typical dosing of ceftriaxone is two grams every day, or two grams twice daily for four consecutive days per week. It is most commonly administered via a PICC line, which has its advantages and disadvantages. On the plus side, it allows patients the convenience of doing their own dosing at home rather than traveling to a doctor's office for each treatment, and it can be more cost effective. The downside is that the PICC is susceptible to infection and must be maintained carefully, typically requiring weekly maintenance by a home health care agency. It can limit activities, and care must be taken not to dislodge it. Insurance does not always cover the insertion of the PICC, which can be costly, and IV antibiotics may need to be continued for several months to upwards of a year.

IV ceftriaxone has been a Godsend for many patients with neurological manifestations of Lyme including the typical Lyme Brain symptoms.

Other cephalosporins include cefuroxime and cefdinir, which are 2nd and 3rd generation cephalosporins, respectively. Cefuroxime is one of the medications recommended in the IDSA guidelines for acute Lyme treatment. Overall, I regard cefdinir as more effective than cefuroxime for my patients; however, I do not see either as being highly efficacious in treating Lyme Brain. Those medications simply do not have good blood-brain barrier penetration.

BICILLIN L-A

The penicillin family of medications is also used to treat the spirochete forms of Lyme, similar to the cephalosporin family. Again, there is one medication in this category that stands out.

Bicillin L-A is a long-acting penicillin that is given by intramuscular injection (IM). The injection is given two to three times weekly (every 72 hours is ideal). In the United States, the standard strength is 1.2 million units per vial. In other countries it may vary. In Australia, for example, it is 0.9 million units per vial, so patients often use more than one vial per dose.

Bicillin itself has been around for a long time and is quite well tolerated. An obvious contraindication to its use is a penicillin allergy. If a patient has previously had a reaction to penicillin with any respiratory involvement, I won't even try Bicillin.

However, I have used Bicillin successfully in patients who as children had reported rashes from penicillin but had not experienced any adverse reactions since. Of course, we err on the side of caution, and if there seems to be any possibility of an anaphylactic reaction, we avoid it at all costs.

Bicillin can cause powerful Herxheimer reactions. Some people Herx after a few days on Bicillin, while others may experience a delayed Herx around day 25. These reactions, which I see more of than actual side effects, are a reflection of how well it works. With more sensitive patients, I might start with half a vial once a week and build up gradually from there.

Bicillin injections are not everyone's favorite activity. Some people tolerate it well and have no problem at all, while others find it uncomfortable. Some hints for making the injection more comfortable are:

❖ Take the vial out of the fridge 30-45 minutes before the injection so that the solution is at room temperature.

❖ Apply lidocaine or Emla cream to the injection site before injecting.

❖ Inject slowly over 1-2 minutes.

❖ Use ice before the injection and a heating pad afterwards. (Some people prefer it the other way around. Try both and see what helps you the most.)

❖ Massage the area afterwards to help disperse the solution throughout the muscle tissue.

I use Bicillin L-A extensively in my practice. It is the medication that my patients tell me "gives them their brain back." Sometimes, if insurance denies coverage for Bicillin, people ask if there is an alternative, and there is. They can take oral amoxicillin, or oral cefuroxime or cefdinir, but neither of those medications is going to give the dramatic improvement in Lyme Brain that Bicillin can potentially give. Most of my patients would take a sore, lumpy bottom over Lyme Brain any day of the week!

Oral amoxicillin is used quite frequently in Lyme treatment, but it just does not have the same power or potency as Bicillin L-A to cross the blood-brain barrier and help with Lyme Brain. Some of my really sensitive patients may start on oral amoxicillin or take it while traveling if the Bicillin shots would be impossible to do, but it is not a medication that I prefer or find highly effective overall.

MINOCYCLINE

Minocycline is in the tetracycline family of antibiotics. While it can be given intravenously, it is typically given orally to Lyme patients. Of all the tetracyclines, minocycline has the greatest penetration of the blood-brain barrier, which makes it a valid choice for patients with neurological symptoms and Lyme Brain. It is reported to have five times greater central nervous system penetration than doxycycline, primarily because it is five times more lipophilic.[1]

The bad news here, and often a limiting factor, is minocycline's side effect profile. It can cause vestibular disturbance leading to dizziness, vertigo, ataxia (loss of control of body movement) and tinnitus. These side effects are more likely to occur in women. In fact, 50-70% of women who are given minocycline experience these side effects and will typically need to stop the medication entirely if they occur.[2]

Minocycline shares some of the other side effects as doxycycline. It can cause sun sensitivity, although it is typically less severe than with doxy. It can also cause some gastrointestinal disturbance although usually less severe than doxy.

All in all, most Lyme doctors still choose doxycycline over minocycline for a cell-wall deficient medication and most certainly in the treatment of acute Lyme disease. Doxycycline is a better medication for treating Borrelia *overall*, while minocycline is a slightly lesser medication *overall*, but still does have better nervous system penetration specifically. The limitation of higher doses of minocycline due to the potential of vestibular disturbance is significant.

I do use minocycline in patients who might be highly sensitive and need a gentler medication to start out with (although I'll typically opt for azithromycin in these cases). I also use it for those who have done well on doxy but side effects make it difficult to continue, and in certain cases, for those where we need as much blood-brain barrier penetration as possible, such as in patients who have a penicillin allergy and cannot do Bicillin L-A injections. Typically, a therapeutic trial is the only way to tell if a patient is going to experience the vestibular side effects of minocycline, but it is important to look out for that. If a patient experiences headache and dizziness as a typical Lyme symptom, it can also be hard to tell if the worsening of those specific symptoms is due to a Herx reaction or the side effects of the medication itself.

Another important consideration about minocycline is its anti-inflammatory properties and its ability to support neural regeneration, which we'll talk about in just a little bit.

DOXYCYCLINE

Doxycycline is still regarded to have some blood-brain barrier penetration although not quite that of minocycline. This is largely because it is lipophilic; that is, it is drawn to fat molecules, which makes it more absorbable. Further, doxy's penetration is also dose-dependent. At 200mg per day, it is considered bacteriostatic (able to halt the progression of infection), while at 400mg per day it is bacteriocidal (able to kill bacteria sufficiently to overcome infection). It is the higher doses that also "push" the medication more effectively into the central nervous system.

Doxycycline does not create the same vestibular disturbances as minocycline, which is a huge advantage. However, the side effects of sun sensitivity and gastrointestinal distress are more severe in doxy than in minocycline. Building up the dose gradually can help the body to adjust and minimize the GI disturbance, but all patients must be very careful to avoid sun exposure. Even a few minutes in the sun can lead to quite severe sunburns and heat rashes. Sunscreen is not a sufficient barrier, so clothing must be worn to cover all exposed skin. People on doxy also need to be careful while driving. I have had many patients burn on the hand that is closest to the window and, hence, sun exposed.

Doxy absorbs better when taken on an empty stomach, but due to the potential gastritis, it is often recommended to be taken with food (food reduces absorption by approximately 20%). This is particularly important when giving the higher doses that we do in Lyme treatment. However, dairy products will reduce its absorption (but I know that you have read The Lyme Diet and cut dairy out of your diet, right?), and minerals taken at the same time, such as calcium, magnesium, iron and zinc, will too.

Overall, doxycycline is one of the key medications we use in treating Lyme disease, both acute and chronic. I do find it helpful to reduce Lyme Brain but not to the extent of medications given via IV or IM routes such as Rocephin and Bicillin.

METRONIDAZOLE AND TINIDAZOLE

Metronidazole and tinidazole are mostly used in Lyme treatment to address and prevent the cyst forms of Borrelia. These two medications are both small and lipophilic, and subsequently, can cross the blood-brain barrier easily. In fact, metronidazole is the standard therapy in medicine for bacterial brain abscesses.

Beyond the cyst forms, research shows that tinidazole has good activity against all three forms of Borrelia, including biofilm colonies.[3]

In fact, the published results were as follows:

"Doxycycline reduced spirochetal structures ~90%, but increased the number of round body forms about twofold. Amoxicillin reduced spirochetal forms by ~85%–90% and round body forms by ~68%, while treatment with metronidazole led to reduction of spirochetal structures by ~90% and round body forms by ~80%. Tigecycline and tinidazole treatment reduced both spirochetal and round body forms by ~80%–90%. When quantitative effects on biofilm-like colonies were evaluated, the five antibiotics reduced formation of these colonies by only

30%–55%. In terms of qualitative effects, only tinidazole reduced viable organisms by ~90%. Following treatment with the other antibiotics, viable organisms were detected in 70%–85% of the biofilm-like colonies."

Let me try to simplify that for you (all numbers signify reductions with the exception of doxycycline increasing round body forms):

	Spirochete	Round body	Eradicated Biofilm
Doxycycline	90%	↑200%	70-85%
Amoxicillin	85-90%	68%	70-85%
Metronidazole	90%	80%	70-85%
Tigecycline	80-90%	80-90%	70-85%
Tinidazole	80-90%	80-90%	90%

Because of the blood-brain barrier penetration of tinidazole, coupled with its ability to impact multiple forms of the Borrelia bacteria and biofilm colonies, tinidazole should be regarded as a key player in chronic Lyme treatment.

Tinidazole can certainly cause quite significant Herx reactions; however, I do believe that reflects its broad-based efficacy. I utilize tinidazole more than metronidazole in my practice, not only because of the research favoring its efficacy against Borrelia, but also because it has far fewer gastrointestinal side effects and is much easier to tolerate for most people. It can make a good contribution towards overcoming Lyme Brain.

MEDICATIONS THAT ARE NOT SO GREAT FOR LYME BRAIN

There are many more antibiotics that are used for Lyme disease than those previously listed. The following are examples of those that do not have superior blood-brain barrier penetration (this is not a complete list—there are hundreds of antibiotics—but these are among the more common ones used in Lyme treatment):

❖ Macrolides—azithromycin, clarithromycin, roxithromycin

❖ Cephalosporins—cefdinir, cefuroxime, cefotaxime, cefixime

❖ Penicillins—amoxicillin, ampicillin

Bear in mind that these medications have some blood-brain barrier penetration. They are just not the best medications for this purpose. Some of you might have experienced dramatic improvement in Lyme Brain from one of more of these medications. This may be explained by their partial penetration, other mechanisms of action such as immune-modulating effects or by the degree of inflammation in the brain regulating how much of the medication can pass (remember we discussed that in highly inflammatory conditions, many more antibiotics will be effective because the inflamed meninges allow for greater passage of molecules into the brain).

Remember also that some Lyme Brain can be caused by infection elsewhere in the body with the overall inflammation being the cause rather than infection in the brain itself. In this case, antibiotics that kill pathogens anywhere in the body could still secondarily help Lyme Brain by reducing overall inflammation.

ANTIBIOTICS USED FOR THE CO-INFECTIONS OF LYME DISEASE

The most common co-infections of Borrelia are Babesia, Bartonella, Ehrlichia—Anaplasma phagocytophilum (HGE) and Human Monocytic Ehrlichia (HME)—and Rickettsia. The two subtypes of Ehrlichia along with Rickettsia species are typically treated with doxycycline, minocycline, azithromycin or rifampin. Therefore, the information given for those medications applies to those particular co-infections. Babesia and Bartonella have more distinct medications so will be discussed separately here.

BARTONELLA MEDICATIONS

Rifampin, in the rifamycin family, is a medication used primarily for Bartonella. It is sometimes used for Anaplasma, especially in patients who cannot tolerate tetracyclines. Even though rifampin is highly lipophilic, it is a large molecule and does not permeate the blood-brain barrier well, except in cases of meningeal inflammation.

The quinolone family of medications does a better job of crossing the blood-brain barrier. They include ciprofloxacin and levofloxacin, which is also used to treat Bartonella. They are moderately lipophilic, relatively small and have low binding to plasma proteins.

Quinolones have good blood-brain barrier penetration even without meningeal inflammation (and remember, while we acknowledge that Lyme is a disease that results in extensive inflammation, there is typically not the level of meningeal inflammation that would be required to allow permeability of all antibiotics).

Therefore, from a Lyme Brain perspective, Levaquin might be a better choice than rifampin. However, we also have to bear in mind other factors with the quinolone family of medications, such as the potential for tendon damage and even rupture. Certain precautions can be taken to prevent it, such as supplementing with magnesium and alpha-lipoic acid, but there is still a risk. As with any Lyme protocol, decisions must be made on an individual basis, in tandem with patients and their Lyme-literate doctors, bearing in mind the risk-benefit relationship of certain decisions.

BABESIA MEDICATIONS

Mepron and Malarone, which contain the active ingredient atovaquone, are two of the more common medications used to treat Babesia. Mepron is pure atovaquone in liquid form, and Malarone is a tablet with atovaquone and proguanil combined.

Atovaquone is highly lipophilic, but it is also extensively bound to plasma proteins. Studies have demonstrated that it is not absorbed into the brain to any appreciable extent making it of limited benefit for "Babesia Lyme Brain."[4] Mepron and Malarone are still the primary medications used for Babesia, and they can be very beneficial overall, but I would always pair or rotate them with something that has better blood-brain barrier penetration such as Riamet/Coartem or Alinia.

Artemether/lumefantrine, marketed under the brand names Riamet and Coartem, may be helpful in addressing the "brain" elements of Babesia due to somewhat better blood-brain barrier penetration than atovaquone. I have seen good changes with this medication, with few side effects and little toxicity. I do weekly three-day pulses of Coartem for the first month of administration, then three days per fortnight (two-week period) thereafter. Typically, in the second month, I will "layer in" another Babesia agent such as an atovoquone-based medication (just not given on the days Coartem is taken) and/or the herbs artemisinin or cryptolepis.

Nitazoxanide (Alinia) is another medication that is less frequently used in Babesia treatment but may be helpful because of its ability to cross the blood-brain barrier. It can also be used when there is atovaquone resistance, which seems to occur more and more these days. Alinia can be challenging because of the gastrointestinal disturbance it can cause, but for those who can tolerate it, it has been effective against Babesia and especially helpful for the brain-related aspects. Alinia may also have activity against cyst forms of Borrelia and other intestinal parasites (its on-label use is infectious diarrhea caused by Cryptosporidium parvum and Giardia lamblia), so it's a good multitasker.

Mefloquine (Larium) is another drug that is somewhat infrequently used in Babesiosis. One of my mentors used Larium extensively, and we saw amazing results in terms of the central nervous system aspects of Babesia (e.g., anxiety, depression, dizziness and head pressure). Larium has something of a questionable reputation due to its ability to cause neuropsychiatric side effects, and to be sure, care must be taken in its use and patients monitored for potential issues. Those with diagnosed neuropsychiatric illness, seizure disorders or cardiac conduction disturbances should avoid Larium. It is reported that mild psychiatric side effects of sleep disturbance, vivid dreams and mood changes occur in 5% to 30% of people. More severe reactions of psychosis or convulsions occur in 1 in 10,000 individuals or less.[5] Interestingly, the milder side effects of sleep disturbance, vivid dreams and mood changes sound very much like some of the symptoms of Babesia, don't they? It can be tricky to discern side effects of the medication from Babesia Herxheimer reactions.

Sulfonamides and trimethoprim are considered to be good agents for blood-brain barrier penetration. They are lipophilic and their molecular size is small. In patients who do not experience sulfa-drug allergy or sensitivity, I have found Bactrim (trimethoprim and sulfamethoxazole combined) to be a good medication for intracellular co-infections such as Babesia and Bartonella, and more effective than trimethoprim alone. While not really a stand-alone medication for either of the co-infections, I often add it to a protocol with an atovaquone-based medication (Mepron or Malarone) or even with Riamet/Coartem to boost the efficacy of the protocol for Babesia, but again, not given on the same days as that medication. (Note: Bactrim should not be given with Rifampin due to adverse drug interactions, and people who are allergic to sulfa drugs cannot take Bactrim.)

REFERENCES

[1] eMed Expert. "eMed Expert Comparisions." *Doxycycline versus minocycline.* http://www.emedexpert.com/compare-meds/doxycycline-vs-minocycline.shtml (accessed 2015).

[2] Sweet, Richard L, and Ronald S Gibbs. *Infectious Diseases of the Female Genital Tract.* 4th. Philadelphia: Lippincott Williams & Wilkins, 2001.

[3] Sapi, Eva, et al. "Evaluation of in-vitro antibiotic susceptibility of different morphological forms of Borrelia burgdorferi." *Infect Drug Resist* 4 (2011): 97-113.

[4] Spencer, C M, and K L Goa. "Atovaquone. A review of its pharmacological properties and therapeutic efficacy in opportunistic infections." *Drugs* 50, no. 1 (1995): 176-96.

[5] Baggish, Aaron L, and David R Hill. "Antiparasitic Agent Atovaquone." *Antimicrob Agents Chemother* 46, no. 5 (May 2002): 1163-1173.

CHAPTER 9

MEDICATIONS THAT REDUCE

INFLAMMATION

———◦✕◦———

MINOCYCLINE AND DOXYCYCLINE

We've already learned that minocycline and doxycycline can benefit Lyme Brain by crossing the blood-brain barrier to help overcome the infection itself. These two medications have an additional benefit: they are known to be anti-inflammatory. Given that inflammation in the central nervous system is a major contributor to Lyme Brain, this is clinically very significant.

Research confirms that tetracyclines inhibit the inflammatory response to the Borrelia spirochete. In a rhesus monkey study, astrocytes and microglia (two different cell types in the central nervous system) were stimulated either with the Borrelia bacteria or one of its outer surface proteins in the presence of doxycycline and minocycline. Both antibiotics significantly reduced the production of tumor necrosis factor-alpha, interleukin 6, and interleukin 8, which are inflammatory markers that are known to be elevated in Lyme disease.[1]

Another rodent study supported those findings and showed that doxycycline had a greater anti-inflammatory effect than minocycline.[2]

Of even further benefit, doxycycline and minocycline are thought to be neuroprotective; that is, they protect cells in the nervous system from damage and degeneration, and even cell death. There are a couple of proposed mechanisms for this. One is the inhibition of microglial activation and dysregulation; the other is a reduction in the reactive oxygen species—"oxidants"—that can damage and destroy neurons. Minocycline and doxycycline can directly scavenge free radicals and modulate enzymes such as nitric oxide synthase and lipoxygenases.

They also appear to reduce excitotoxins—including glutamate—in the brain.[3] Excitotoxins are a class of chemicals, usually amino acids, which overstimulate neuron production. Some excitotoxins come from the diet. Well-known ones include monosodium glutamate (MSG) and artificial sweeteners such as aspartame. In other cases, increases in excitotoxins such as glutamate occur without any outside influences. Either way, they are considered to be neurotoxic and highly detrimental to the nervous system, and minocycline can help to reduce them. Disclaimer: Please do not take this as license to ingest MSG or artificial sweeteners. All Lyme patients should avoid them like the plague, even those taking minocycline!

In the realm of neuroprotection, minocycline is thought to be more effective than doxycycline.[4]

These findings are significant not only for Lyme disease patients, but also in cases of stroke, Parkinson's disease, CNS trauma and other neurodegenerative diseases.

All in all, the anti-inflammatory and neuroprotective benefits of minocycline and doxycycline combined with their moderate blood-brain barrier penetration make them good medication choices for Lyme patients.

LOW DOSE NALTREXONE

Low dose naltrexone (LDN) is another medication that can have anti-inflammatory effects in the body. In fact, low dose naltrexone has several beneficial impacts. Not only is it immune modulating, but it can help balance out moods and sleep patterns too.

Low dose naltrexone (LDN) is used in many illnesses and syndromes, among them Lyme disease, fibromyalgia, chronic fatigue syndrome, multiple sclerosis, autism, rheumatoid arthritis, HIV and cancer. Because it works to balance the immune system, any condition that involves immune dysregulation may benefit from LDN.

Some people have heard that naltrexone is a substance that doctors give to drug addicts to get them off opioid drugs, such as morphine and heroin, by binding with the opioid receptors and blocking the drugs from being able to attach. It is true that it functions this way, but that is a synthetic medication that is given at high doses in that context.

LDN is a very low dose of a compounded form of naltrexone, which means that instead of 50mg to 300mg being given, the dose ranges are from 1mg to 4.5mg. Instead of being a prefabricated commercial medication, it is a pure form of naltrexone that is encapsulated by a compounding pharmacy (or in some cases, put into a transdermal application).

LDN works by providing a very weak binding effect on the opioid receptors in the brain. This causes two things to happen. Firstly, enkephalins are released, or "up-regulated," in response to that weak binding. Enkephalins are immune chemicals that help modulate immune function. That means that they can strengthen weak immune function and down-regulate overactive immune function in the case of autoimmune disease.

The second effect is an increased release of endorphins. Endorphins are the feel-good chemicals. For many people, more endorphins result in greater energy, enhanced mood and reduced pain levels.

LDN has very few side effects. Some people report some difficulty sleeping in the first week or so, which typically resolves spontaneously. I have found that starting at 1.5mg and incrementally working up to 4.5mg dramatically reduces the incidence of sleep disturbance that is possible in the early days of LDN. I suggest starting with 1.5mg (1 capsule) for 3–4 nights, then going up to 3mg (2 capsules) for a few nights, and finally, up to 4.5mg (3 capsules) thereafter. Some people feel better at a lower dose and choose to stay at 1.5mg or 3mg indefinitely. One does not offset the benefit by taking a lower dose. If you feel better at that dose, then it's a better dose for you.

There are a few cautions with LDN. For example, a patient with Hashimoto's thyroiditis with low thyroid function may need to monitor their thyroid medication carefully, as when the thyroid starts functioning better after the LDN, the regular dose of medication may become too much. The lowest possible dose of LDN (1.5mg) is a good starting point in these cases.

LDN should not be taken by those on narcotic pain medications or by transplant recipients.

LDN can function not only as an anti-inflammatory, but because it increases endorphins, it can have antidepressant benefits, too.[5] Given that Lyme Brain and depression are quite good friends, alleviating depression is an important consideration in treatment.

In my practice, I have found that LDN is not effective to regulate mood and reduce pain for everyone. The people for whom it works love it, but there are some who do not see great benefit and discontinue taking it. With a reasonably low cost and side effect profile, I believe it is worth a 30-day trial.

REFERENCES

[1] Bernardino, A L, D Kaushal, and M T Philipp. "The antibiotics doxycycline and minocycline inhibit the inflammatory responses to the Lyme disease spirochete Borrelia burgdorferi." *J Infect Dis* 199, no. 9 (May 2009): 1379-88.

[2] Leite, L M, et al. "Anti-inflammatory properties of doxycycline and minocycline in experimental models: an in vivo and in vitro comparative study." *Inflammapharmacology* 19, no. 2 (April 2011): 99-110.

[3] Plane, Jennifer M, Yan Shen, David E Pleasure, and Wenbin Deng. "Prospects for Minocycline Neuroprotection." *Arch Neurol* 67, no. 12 (December 2010): 1442-1448.

[4] Leite, L M, et al. "Anti-inflammatory properties." 99-110.

[5] Brown, N, and J Panksepp. "Low-dose naltrexone for disease prevention and quality of life." *Med Hypotheses* 72, no. 3 (March 2009): 333-7.

CHAPTER 10

MEDICATIONS THAT INFLUENCE

BRAIN FUNCTION

—◇—

When we consider the range of medications that can be used to stabilize the neurological, cognitive and psychoemotional functions of Lyme patients, there are many options, ranging from stimulants to anti-seizure medications.

For the sake of organization, I have grouped these into three major categories:

1. Medications that stabilize neurological function

2. Medications that stabilize mood

3. Medications that support cognition

Some patients may need one medication from each category, and many will not take any of them. Some may find them to be lifesaving while others may not experience any benefit. There is no guarantee that any of the medications mentioned will help Lyme Brain. In many cases, the only thing that will truly help Lyme Brain is treating the Lyme infection and inflammation itself. However, sometimes, some supportive therapy along the way can provide symptomatic relief. We must also remember that some people have coexisting psychiatric and psychological issues that are not caused by Lyme disease, issues that would be present whether or not they had Lyme. Perhaps Lyme disease made them worse, but we must also take care not to blame everything on Lyme and address other issues as we identify them.

Since I am naturopathically trained and oriented, I help my patients naturally whenever possible. However, there are definitely times when stabilizing neurological function is necessary. Support with an antidepressant can give enough relief *while the underlying cause is being addressed* and give the brain a helping hand through cognition support or neurotransmitter balancing. I try to do this using natural means, and the next section is dedicated to that, but there are certainly times where I refer out to other physicians for assistance in stabilizing my patients.

Most of the following medications listed have side effects and interactions with other medications. To list all of them is beyond the scope of this book, but bear in mind that though a medication may sound great on paper, in reality, it may create unmanageable side effects or secondary problems. That is where the sound clinical judgment of prescribing doctors is crucial.

Many of the medications used to ameliorate issues related to Lyme disease have other on-label uses, such as epilepsy, bipolar disorder, Alzheimer's and dementia. Sadly, there is just not enough research on the neuropsychiatric aspects of Lyme disease with a view towards developing medications that specifically address the problem. So for now, doctors seek out solutions based on the medications that help similar symptoms falling under other diagnoses.

I also want to differentiate between Lyme Brain, which we tend to think of as the cognitive deficits such as memory loss and brain fog that come from Lyme disease; and the more severe psychiatric manifestations such as bipolar disorder, severe depression or anxiety, obsessive-compulsive disorder, panic attacks and psychosis. For the majority of this book, I will discuss Lyme Brain and refer mostly to the brain fog/memory/concentration issues that ensue, including mild to moderate anxiety and depression. I'll give an overview of other medications because they might be relevant for many people, and for others, there is an extensive overlap of symptoms.

So back to our medication categories. Again, this is by no means an exhaustive list. Instead, it is a brief overview of some of the possibilities. Please discuss this further with your Lyme-literate physician, neurologist or psychiatrist.

MEDICATIONS THAT STABILIZE NEUROLOGICAL FUNCTION

ANTI-SEIZURE MEDICATIONS

A certain percentage of patients with Lyme disease experience seizures or seizure-like activity. This can be due to inflammatory changes in the brain, lack of oxygen and blood, and metabolic issues such as high or low blood sugar. When true epilepsy develops as a result of chronic infection, anti-epilepsy drugs can be very successful in stabilizing them. However, it is estimated that about 25% of patients with seizures do not respond to epilepsy drugs and do not have actual epilepsy but instead have non-epileptic seizures.[1] Put simply, they have seizures but do not have epilepsy. I have seen many cases of seizures and seizure-like activity resolve completely during Lyme treatment without the need for ongoing anti-seizure medication. That tells me that by clearing the infection, the trigger for the seizures is removed and the nervous system can be calmed and stabilized once more.

There are many anti-seizure medications. Examples are carbamazepine (Tegratol), lamotrigine (Lamictal), gapapentin (Neurontin), valproic acid (Depakene), divalproex sodium (Depakote) and phenytoin (Dilantin). This is just a brief account of a long list of possibilities; there are over forty different anti-seizure medications. A prescription is based on the individual case, which takes into account age, type and frequency of seizures, lifestyle and the possibility of pregnancy in women.

While it's obvious to state that anti-seizure medications are used to stabilize neurological function and prevent seizures, there are also off-label uses for them. In Lyme patients, certain anti-seizure medications can be used to reduce or prevent pain, and to reduce neuropathy.

One of the most commonly prescribed medications in this category is pregabalin, or Lyrica. It is actually used more for neuropathy and pain than it is for actual seizures. Its applications include diabetic neuropathy, nerve pain following spinal cord injury or damage to peripheral nerves, fibromyalgia pain and nerve pain caused by shingles. In fact, Lyrica was the first medication to be approved for use in fibromyalgia in 2007.

For some Lyme patients, Lyrica makes a significant dent in chronic neuropathic pain and generalized neuralgia. In reports from my patients, it is not effective for everyone and in some can give unwanted side effects. Some people find benefit from it for their generalized anxiety. Despite some side effects, including dizziness, drowsiness, visual disturbance, weight gain, and tremors (amongst many others), it may still be a better option than narcotic pain medications or benzodiazepines with their significant risk of dependence.

ANTIPSYCHOTIC MEDICATIONS

Antipsychotics are primarily used for psychosis in schizophrenia and bipolar disorder. These medications are categorized as major tranquilizers or neuroleptics and function to reduce symptoms such as delusions and hallucinations. Well-known examples of antipsychotics include risperidone (Risperdal), quietiapine (Seroquel) and haloperidol (Haldol).

Peer reviewed research has shown a link between schizophrenia and Lyme disease.[2,3,4] Furthermore, regions with high rates of Lyme disease have significant correlations with regions with high rates of schizophrenia.[5]

There is also some research on the seasonal correlations between schizophrenia and Lyme.[6] In the United States, Japan and Europe, the births of people who later develop schizophrenia mirror the seasonal distribution of ticks nine months earlier. How close or relevant the association is may not be crystal clear, but it is an interesting hypothesis to consider.

A person suffering from Lyme disease may manifest schizophrenic tendencies as a result of the infectious process in their brain. The co-infection Bartonella can also cause these severe psychiatric manifestations. Hence, antipsychotic medications may have a place in Lyme treatment where Borrelia infection is the underlying cause of schizophrenia and bipolar disorders. They may also have a place in treating obsessive-compulsive disorder, Tourette's syndrome, post-traumatic stress disorder, personality disorders and agitation associated with dementia. They have been used occasionally to reduce aggressive behavior and irritability in children and adolescents with autism.

Of course, not all psychiatric disorders are caused by Borrelia or Bartonella infection, so a thorough work up and evaluation must be done. Having said that, given that chronic infection is a possible cause, and given an infection is treatable, where psychiatric disorders such as schizophrenia are considered permanent (with the goal being suppression of adverse manifestations), we can only hope that every person with a psychiatric illness such as this has the opportunity to get evaluated for Lyme. Imagine how sad it would be for a child to go through life on a major tranquilizer drug when the proper diagnosis and treatment of Lyme disease may have been able to circumvent it.

MOOD STABILIZERS

Mood stabilizers are medications that balance out the shifts in moods that come with bipolar disorder. By shifts in mood, I don't mean that one minute you're pretty happy and the next minute you're grumpy (that is most Lyme patients I speak to, by their own report!). Bipolar disorder is a true psychiatric illness categorized by periods of severe depression punctuated by episodes of mania. Suicidal tendencies are common. Mood-stabilizing medications can also be used in schizoaffective disorder and borderline personality disorder.

Lithium is the classic and best-known mood stabilizer, with good efficacy in preventing manic episodes. It is also sometimes used in combination with antidepressants in unipolar depression (depression without manic episodes). It is thought to work by reducing norepinephrine and increasing serotonin synthesis.

The pharmacological lithium is either in carbonate or citrate form. As we will discuss in the section on natural solutions for Lyme Brain, a different form of lithium called lithium orotate can be used as a nutritional supplement and can be helpful for supporting brain function.

Since the medication lithium can have significant effects on sodium and water balance in the body, regular blood work must be done to monitor for signs of dehydration. Blood levels of the medication must also be checked to make sure the effective dose is maintained without reaching toxic levels.

Antipsychotics and anti-seizure meds are also used as mood stabilizers in some cases. There is an overlap with these medications and categories, so it is quite difficult to divide them into neat and tidy sections.

MEDICATIONS THAT BALANCE MOOD

ANTIDEPRESSANT MEDICATIONS

Depression is a common occurrence in Lyme patients. Many Lyme patients who I have encountered realize that there's a close association between depression and what they call Lyme Brain; that is, their cognitive function is closely tied to their emotional state. It is unclear whether this is cause or effect in either direction, or whether it so happens that when they have more inflammation in their bodies, such as when they are Herxing, both symptoms are exacerbated. Either way, it is a double whammy for the patient and can put them in a hole that can be hard to climb out of.

Many patients have been told that all their Lyme symptoms are related to depression. They are depressed; therefore, they experience these debilitating and diverse systemic symptoms. In my experience, it is usually the exact opposite—they experience these horrible symptoms and interruptions to their life as they know it, and subsequently, they become depressed. That is a fairly normal and natural human reaction.

Remember earlier when we talked a little about depression and anxiety, and I mentioned that there are two mechanisms at work: one is the normal, natural human reaction to the experience of chronic illness, pain, inflammation, fatigue and so on. The second is the infections themselves, which cause disturbances in the neurological system that lead to inflammatory processes, neurotransmitter imbalances, toxic stress and other distinct physiological process that mess with brain chemistry and mood regulation.

Yes, it is all in your head, but not in the way you've been accused by not-very-compassionate or understanding doctors. The infection is in your head, the inflammation is in your head, the neurotransmitter imbalance is in your head—they are all very real things that are going on in your head. They can be changed with the appropriate treatment and you can recover. Please take heart.

The other point I should make here is that there is a difference between the psychiatric disorders of dysthymia, a milder form of depression, reactive depression, which is a natural response to a bad and painful set of circumstances, and major depressive disorder. Many people suffer from major depressive disorder and did so even before their Lyme diagnosis and potentially even before their illness with Lyme disease. It is a very real and serious psychiatric disorder that typically requires mood-stabilizing medication.

So while I make the distinction that people who suffer from major depressive disorder will likely need antidepressant medications to be stable, even those with a milder depression and reactive depression may benefit. Subsequently, there may be a role for antidepressant medications in a subset of Lyme patients. This by no means implies that depression is the cause of all their health issues, but if depression is secondary to the chronic infectious process, there are times when short- to medium-term use of an antidepressant is beneficial to get them through the most challenging times. In some cases, it can be lifesaving.

Some antidepressants are also approved for use in chronic pain and neuropathic pain. This is why they can be prescribed for fibromyalgia syndrome and why they might also be relevant to Lyme patients, even those who are not depressed.

There are a few categories of antidepressant medications. A very well-known category is the SSRI group, or the selective serotonin reuptake inhibitors. These medications function by encouraging the recycling of serotonin rather than the discarding of it. That way, the serotonin molecules get reused, and if there is a shortage of serotonin, it will optimize what is there. Examples of SSRIs include paroxetine (Paxil), sertraline (Zoloft), citalopram (Celexa) and fluoxetine (Prozac).

There are also serotonin-norepinephrine reuptake inhibitors (SNRI), which as the name suggests, encourage the reutilization of both serotonin and norepinephrine. Serotonin is a more calming, soothing neurotransmitter while norepinephrine is more stimulating. Some people find SSRIs by themselves too sedating and do better with this dual approach. Also, if both the serotonin and norepinephrine pathways are depleted or under-functioning, an SNRI will provide more comprehensive relief. Examples are duloxetine (Cymbalta), desvenlafaxine (Pristiq) and venlafaxine (Effexor).

Buproprion (Wellbutrin) is an antidepressant that is used extensively, partially because it does not cause unwanted sexual side effects and weight gain. It is a norepinephrine and dopamine reuptake inhibitor, so it works on two of the pathways in the brain but *not* the serotonin pathway. This medication can be beneficial for many, especially since dopamine is associated with the brain's reward and pleasure responses as well as cognition.

Another somewhat older group of antidepressant medications are the tricyclics. These were the first antidepressant medications to act on both serotonin and norepinephrine; however, they also can interact with other chemical messengers in the neurological system, which gives them a higher potential for side effects. Some tricyclics are approved for use in pain, and some are used as sleep aids. For the most part, the newer generation antidepressants have taken over their use. Examples of tricyclics are amitriptyline (Elavil), imipramine (Tofranil), clomipramine (Anafranil) and desipramine (Norpramin).

The last category is monoamine oxidase inhibitors (MAOI), which inhibit the monoamine oxidase enzymes. The overall goal is similar to other classes of neurotransmitters: to keep more serotonin, norephinephrine, epinephrine and dopamine in the brain. The mechanism is what makes the difference. Historically, MAOIs have come with dietary concerns, especially with cheese and other high-tyramine foods. The premise is that the enzymes in the medications interfere with the ability to fully break down the tyramines in foods, which can lead to a hypertensive crisis. Examples of high-tyramine foods include liver, alcohol, many cheeses, aged pickled meats, chocolate, Vegemite/Marmite—in fact, anything that's been pickled, fermented, smoked, aged or marinated. That's okay, because again, I know you're all following *The Lyme Diet* and these foods aren't even in your repertoire (however, even healthy fermented foods like kimchi and kefir might prove problematic for people on MAOIs). That historical research and all the food restrictions are being challenged now, plus there are newer MAOIs coming out that are approved for use without dietary restrictions, such as seleginine (often used in Parkinson's disease) and rasagiline.[7] Both of these work more on the dopamine pathways than the serotonin/norepinephrine ones.

While I am not delving into all the possible side effects of all the medications mentioned (that would make for a very long and boring book!), I do want to make the point that while antidepressants can be life changing and a Godsend, they do not work well for everyone. Some have significant side effects; some simply do not do the job; and some leave people worse off when they stop taking them. Some argue that while many of these medications work by preventing the "throwing out" of neurotransmitters and encouraging what's there to be recycled and reused, if there is a fundamental shortage of that neurotransmitter in the first place, all the recycling in the world won't make the body produce more. Some also believe that the constant recycling can negatively impact the body's ability to produce its own neurotransmitters. Another option is to do amino acid therapy, which involves taking amino acids to provide raw materials so that the body can produce more of its own neurotransmitters. This will be explained in more detail in the next section, but I wanted to introduce the idea here.

ANTI-ANXIETY MEDICATIONS

Anxiety is one of the most common psychological aspects of Lyme and, in my experience, even more so than depression. Again, it is a double-edged sword. The chronic infections in the body can create anxiety as a symptom, just as real as joint pain is a symptom. Then there is the anxiety that comes secondary to the illness: the anxiety of not knowing when (or if) you will be healthy again, if you can support your family or take care of your children, or if you will experience your previous quality of life again. There are many medications that can have anti-anxiety properties.

Many of the antidepressant medications discussed earlier can also reduce anxiety, and so these may be tried first. These include the SSRIs, tricyclics, MAOIs and some of the newer atypical antidepressants.

Antidepressant medications have a lower potential for dependence and abuse than other options such as benzodiazepines, but they are also slower acting. They can take several weeks to have any effect and do not give the immediate calming effect of some of the other medications. In the midst of a panic attack, Xanax is going to work more immediately and effectively but not without its own risks and adverse effects. The most common antidepressants prescribed for anxiety are Prozac, Zoloft, Celexa, Paxil and Lexapro.

Antihistamines are often used for anxiety and sleep issues for their calming and sedating effects. Diphenhydramine, hydroxyzine and doxylamine are some examples in this category. Brand names that might be more familiar include Unisom, Benadryl and NyQuil. These are more likely to be self-prescribed and administered by patients, because they are available over-the-counter. In my experience, a physician is less likely to suggest these options than they are to prescribe an antidepressant or anxiolytic medication. The calming effect of most of these over-the-counter medications is secondary (the reduction in allergy symptoms and sleep promotion is primary) and may feel more like a drowsy, drugged feeling than a true anxiety reduction while leaving other cognitive aspects intact. Still, there is a place for simple and inexpensive interventions such as these, in particular, where nighttime anxiety is preventing or disturbing sleep. Although these medications can be psychologically habit forming, true addiction potential is not a concern.

Speaking of off-label uses for medications, beta-blockers, which are typically prescribed for high blood pressure and cardiovascular issues, have also been used for anxiety. One of their mechanisms of action is to reduce norepinephrine, which is involved in the fight-or-flight response. These medications can calm symptoms of anxiety, in particular, physical symptoms such as racing heart rate, flushing, sweaty palms and tremors. Of course, people with low blood pressure should not take beta-blockers, and for those with asthma, they are not recommended. Propran-olol (Inderal), one of the beta-blockers often prescribed for this purpose, can be helpful for more acute situations such as social anxiety, public speaking or a stress-ful event. Atenolol (Tenormin) is a little longer-acting with fewer immediate side effects but can cause rebound increases in blood pressure when discontinued.

Benzodiazepines are the primary category of anti-anxiety medications. They act as sedatives and tranquilizers. Common ones are lorazepam (Ativan), clonazepam (Klonopin), diazepam (Valium) and alprazolam (Xanax).

These medications seem to be prescribed fairly freely by many physicians and psychiatrists. They work well and quickly for relieving anxiety. However, they are not without their issues.

Firstly, there can be significant interactions when taken with certain other antide-pressants and nervous system depressants such as Benadryl. In combination with alcohol or prescription painkillers, they can provoke a dangerous response and be life threatening.

Secondly, they can foster true physical dependence. Sporadic and minimal dosing is best. People with a history of substance abuse may be more at risk of dependence.

Thirdly, they have side effects that can impact one's cognitive function (less anxiety but more Lyme Brain) and can make driving or operating any equip-ment quite dangerous.

I have excluded certain side effects of many of the aforementioned medications because side effect lists are lengthy and certainly have much individual variance in how the effects can manifest. It's not that the other medications don't have their issues. However, since the benzodiazepines have such significant effects, I feel I must specifically point them out. Here is a list of possible effects:[8]

- ❖ Drowsiness, lack of energy

- ❖ Clumsiness, slow reflexes

- ❖ Slurred speech

- ❖ Confusion and disorientation

- ❖ Depression

- ❖ Dizziness, lightheadedness

- ❖ Impaired thinking and judgment

❖ Memory loss, forgetfulness

❖ Nausea, stomach upset

❖ Blurred vision

❖ Rebound insomnia

Don't many of those side effects sound like Lyme Brain? These medications are potent and powerful, and one of the results of taking them could be symptoms that mimic Lyme Brain, the very effects you're trying to overcome.

I will never forget one particular patient I worked with who had been given Xanax for a short period of time to help her sleep. When she went off it, the rebound insomnia was so severe that she had only slept 1-2 hours a night for months on end.

I do understand that some Lyme sufferers have such debilitating anxiety that they simply cannot function day-to-day without anxiolytic, sedative medication. Some Lyme patients have other symptoms that are intolerable without these medications such as skin crawling or "wanting to jump out of one's skin." I also understand that many have tried other options with no positive results and have resorted to these medications through sheer desperation. As with anything, there is a time and place for these medications. I just want to highlight some of the potential risks for those who might have mild to moderate anxiety as well as other treatment options that might have fewer risks and adverse effects.

Buspirone (brand name BuSpar) is a newer anti-anxiety drug that acts as a tranquilizer, increasing both serotonin and dopamine in the brain. It is also fairly slow-acting, taking a couple of weeks to take effect, but it does have the benefits over the older style anti-anxiety meds of not being as sedating, not compromising cognitive function, and not having the same addiction potential and issues with withdrawal. Given the major issues with benzodiazepines in terms of dependence and withdrawal difficulties, BuSpar might be a better option to try first.

MEDICATIONS THAT SUPPORT COGNITION

STIMULANTS

Typically thought of as medications for attention deficit hyperactivity disorders (ADHD), stimulants have been used to increase arousal, focus and concentration in other people without that specific diagnosis. Stimulants can be amphetamine stimulants, such as Adderall, Dexedrine and Vyvance, or they can be methylphenidate stimulants such as Focalin, Ritalin and Concerta. Both increase the transmission of electrical and chemical signals throughout the central nervous system by increasing both norepinephrine and dopamine, and both come in short-acting and long-acting forms. Amphetamine stimulants prolong the *action* of both norepinephrine and dopamine in the brain, but they also increase the *amount* of them as well. Methylphenidate stimulants prolong the *activity* of norepinephrine and dopamine but do not actually increase their production. Amphetamine stimulants also appear to have slightly more abuse potential than the methylphenidate stimulants.

NOREPINEPHRINE REUPTAKE INHIBITORS

Strattera, a non-stimulant, is in the category of medications used to boost cognition and address ADHD, and is classified as a norepinephrine reuptake inhibitor. Norepinephrine is a brain neurotransmitter that has a stimulating affect. Low norepinephrine can contribute to a dull mood, lack of focus and concentration, and general under arousal of the brain. A reuptake inhibitor will increase levels by minimizing the recycling and removal of a substance, so a norepinephrine reuptake inhibitor aims to increase the amount of that particular neurotransmitter, giving the patient benefits to cognitive function and mood. This type of therapy does not have the abuse and dependence potential of the stimulants, so it can be beneficial without as many risks and adverse effects.

ACETYLCHOLINESTERASE INHIBITORS

Acetylcholine is another neurotransmitter that can be influenced with medication. The mechanism of these medications is to inhibit the enzyme that breaks down the acetylcholine. Examples are rivastigmine, galantamine and donepezil.

There are several different applications for these medications. They can be used to treat Alzheimer's disease and dementia, neuropsychiatric symptoms such as apathy, and cognitive deficits, mostly in memory and learning. Since acetylcholine is a neurotransmitter that plays a role in cognitive function, increasing the levels of it in the brain can improve cognition. It is also used in this capacity in schizophrenia.

Acetylcholinesterase inhibitors have also been used to prolong REM sleep but with mixed results.

NMDA RECEPTOR ANTAGONISTS

Memantine (brand name Namenda) is a slightly different class of medication but, like the acetylcholinesterase inhibitors, has been used to address cognitive and memory issues related to Alzheimer's and related disorders. It works by blocking the activity of glutamate. In normal levels, glutamate aids in memory and learning, but if too high, it can cause excitotoxicity and kill nerve cells. There are cases where this medication has been helpful for Lyme patients in supporting cognitive function.

WAKEFULNESS-PROMOTING AGENTS

Modafinil (brand names Provigil and Modavigil) and the related armodafinil (brand name Nuvigil) are medications that fit into this category. Approved uses are to treat the sleepiness that results from sleep apnea and wakefulness disorders such as narcolepsy. Off-label, they have been used by students and executives to promote alertness, as well as individuals who have delayed sleep schedules causing daytime drowsiness. Jet lag, post-chemo brain fog and Lyme Brain could all potentially benefit from these types of medications. The medications can cause a boost in working memory, spatial memory, executive function and attention.

—————⋈—————

All these medications must be prescribed and managed by physicians, neurologists, psychiatrists and other practitioners who are familiar with their dosing schedules, side effects and medication interactions. As with everything in Lyme treatment, what works for one person might not work for another, and for each individual, their needs will change over time. There is a time and place for everything, and there is no shame in seeking out psychiatric help when it is needed.

REFERENCES

[1] Thadani, Vijay. "2011 Lyme and Tick Borne-Diseases National Conference." *Lyme and Tick-borne Diseases Research Center*. October 1-2, 2011. http://www.columbia-lyme.org/research/scientific.html.

[2] Bar, K J, T Jochum, F Hager, W Meissner, and H Sauer. "Painful hallucinations and somatic delusions in a patient with the possible diagnosis of neuroborreliosis." *Clin J Pain* 21, no. 4 (July-August 2005): 362-3.

[3] Roelcke, U, W Barnett, E Wilder-Smith, D Sigmund, and W Hacke. "Untreated neuroborreliosis: Bannwarth's syndrome evolving into acute schizophrenia-like psychosis. A case report." *J Neurol* 239, no. 3 (1992): 129-31.

[4] Fallon, B A, and J A Nields. "Lyme disease: a neuropsychiatric illness." *Am J Psychiatry* 151, no. 11 (November 1994): 1571-83.

[5] Brown Jr., J S. "Geographic correlation of schizophrenia to ticks and tick-borne encephalitis." *Schizophr Bull* 20, no. 4 (1994): 755-75.

[6] Fritzsche, M. "Seasonal correlation of sporadic schizophrenia to Ixodes ticks and Lyme borreliosis." *Int J Health Geogr* 1, no. 1 (2002): 2.

[7] McCabe-Sellers, Beverly J, Cathleen G Staggs, and Margaret L Bogle. "Tyramine in foods and monoamine oxidase inhibitor drugs: A crossroad where medicine, nutrition, pharmacy, and food industry converge." *Journal of Food Composition and Analysis* 19 (2006): S58-S65.

[8] Smith, Melinda, Lawrence Robinson, and Jeanne Segal. "Anxiety Medication: What You Need to Know About Anti-Anxiety Drugs." *HELPGUIDE.ORG*. January 2016. http://www.helpguide.org/articles/anxiety/anxiety-medication.htm.

SECTION 3:

NATURAL APPROACHES
TO LYME BRAIN

C H A P T E R   1 1

INTRODUCTION

So far we've discussed various medications and how they might help Lyme Brain. Now let's turn to some natural approaches—herbs, supplements, amino acids and essential oils—which can make a difference and potentially be as effective as medications without many of the side effects.

We talked in the first section about some of the main causes of Lyme Brain—the pathogens themselves, the inflammatory cascade created by the infections, toxins and neurotransmitter imbalances. Let's look at those specific areas first, and then we'll look at some general recommendations. At the risk of repeating myself, I'll point out again that this is just a sampling of options with which I've typically had the most experience and from which I've found the most benefit. I realize that there are other helpful options, but it is impossible to cover the hundreds of supplements and herbs on the market that are being used in Lyme treatment. I am also focusing on the things that impact brain function specifically, more than the totality of Lyme symptoms.

To help prevent overwhelm as you read through this section, I have also made a list in the Products and Protocols section with some of my favorite specific supplements, and in particular, products that combine these nutrients well in consolidated formulas.

CHAPTER 12

ANTIMICROBIALS

—➤✕◄—

GARLIC

Garlic might be one of the world's oldest medicines. It is supportive of the immune system and the cardiovascular system (acting as a blood thinner), and has antimicrobial properties, amongst many other things. Garlic's main constituent is allicin, which is known to be able to cross the blood-brain barrier, making it a good option for central nervous system infections. It can also assist in overcoming parasitic infections in the gut, and more systemically, mycoplasma and Candida.

One of the challenges is producing garlic supplements that maintain the active levels of allicin. In that sense, eating raw garlic might seem the preferred way to get the goodness right away, but to get sufficient amounts would require a lot of garlic, and that might be upsetting for the digestive system (and for family members nearby!).

In general, freeze-dried supplements may be the best option to preserve the active constituents. Another brand I like a lot is Allimax, which utilizes a fancy extraction process that ensures 100% allicin content per capsule. They also offer a professional grade product called AlliMed, which contains the same extract, just in a higher dosage per capsule. Their liquid extracts are great for kids, too.

I have also just released a fresh garlic extract under the RestorMedicine label that can be combined with any other antimicrobials.

ANDROGRAPHIS

Widely used in Lyme treatment, Andrographis paniculata is one of the most valuable herbs we have in our toolbox. It is a very bitter herb; in fact, it is known as the "King of Bitters." Historically, it was used to treat syphilis, another spirochetal infection, as well as parasites.

It has three main roles in Lyme treatment: 1) anti-spirochetal activity, which means that it can help to reduce the pathogen load in the body; 2) supporting the body's own immune system to fight infection more efficiently. It can help reduce some of the symptoms of Lyme, including joint pain and cardiovascular symptoms, and I have definitely seen it help cognitive symptoms; and 3) protecting against inflammation-mediated neurodegeneration. This means that it actually helps protect the brain from the effects of inflammation, and because inflammation is one of the major causative factors in Lyme Brain, this is a very good thing!

It has this ability because it does cross the blood-brain barrier and can accumulate at significant levels in the central nervous system—the brain, spinal cord and cerebrospinal fluid.

Andrographis is a favorite herb of Stephen Buhner, and he says:

> *"Andrographis is perhaps the best primary herb to use in the treatment of Lyme disease. It is anti-spirochetal, enhances immune function, protects the heart muscle, is anti-inflammatory (helping with arthritic symptoms), crosses the blood/brain barrier where it is active both as an anti-spirochetal and calming agent; enhances liver function and protects the liver; helping clear infection from the body."*[1]

An herb that crosses the blood-brain barrier easily *and* kills spirochetes *and* protects the brain against inflammation? That sounds like a great choice for people with Lyme Brain! I have used andrographis for several years as part of my Lyme Support Formula and have seen good results with it.

POLYGONUM CUSPIDATUM

Polygonum cuspidatum, more commonly known as Japanese knotweed, is a plant that boasts similar benefits to andrographis. It is antimicrobial, anti-inflammatory and protects the brain against the harmful effects of inflammation and neurotoxins.

Japanese knotweed contains resveratrol, both in the cis- and trans- forms. Resveratrol is a potent antioxidant and, for this reason, is used to prevent and treat degenerative neurological disease and cardiovascular disease.

Japanese knotweed crosses the blood-brain barrier easily; hence, it contributes to fighting neurological Lyme as well as reducing inflammation in the brain and protecting brain cells against degeneration.

Polygonum is known for its tenacious nature and its far-reaching effects within the body. It enhances blood flow, and for this reason, it can venture deep into tissues and carry other herbs and supplements into areas where they are needed but may not have reached by themselves. Such "driver" or "carrier" herbs can be very valuable in illnesses such as Lyme, where the spirochetes drive themselves deep and can be hard to access by antimicrobials of any kind.

Fo-Ti, or Polygonum multiflora, is a close relative of Japanese knotweed. It is actually Chinese knotweed and is also used in Lyme treatment with the same benefits as Japanese knotweed.

CAT'S CLAW

Cat's claw, aka Uncaria tomentosa, is another herb that crosses the blood-brain barrier and is used extensively in Lyme treatment. I use cat's claw as part of my Lyme Support Formula (along with guaiacum, andrographis, olive leaf extract and Japanese knotweed), and find it to be a very valuable herb.

By crossing the blood-brain barrier, cat's claw can help in the fight against Lyme Brain by overcoming the spirochetes as well as by modulating the immune system—boosting a weakened system or calming an overactive one. Research has shown it to increase natural killer cells, which are cells in the immune system that play a large role in hunting down and killing foreign pathogens.

It also has anti-inflammatory and anodyne (pain relieving) effects that add to its benefit. Several of the active constituents of cat's claw are strongly neuro-protective, preventing neuronal cell death.

One point of confusion with cat's claw is the conflict between TOA-free and regular cat's claw. By nature, cat's claw contains a high percentage of alkaloids, and these are some of its most significant constituents. It is said that one of the alkaloids, the tetracyclic oxindole alkaloids (TOA), work against the pentacyclic oxindole alkaloids (POA), thus making the herb less effective in its natural form. Subsequently, products have been developed and branded without the TOAs and only contain the POAs. Examples are samento and Prima Uña de Gato.

In my experience, I have seen great efficacy when using the inner bark of cat's claw (TOAs and all), and I do not feel concerned about the TOA element. I like cat's claw as an overall antimicrobial and have seen it greatly benefit people with Lyme Brain.

TEASEL ROOT

Teasel root, or Dipsacus sylvestris, is one of my favorite herbs for Lyme disease treatment, and I use it extensively. The following is based more on my personal experience of it crossing the blood-brain barrier than from solid research.

Teasel root is well known for its benefit to the musculoskeletal system. It is great for cases of Lyme that impact connective tissues, and it helps with muscle and joint pain, and inflammation.

I have seen teasel root cause significant Herxheimer reactions—typically involving Lyme Brain symptoms—even at small doses. This leads me to believe that it has at least some central nervous system penetration. I also see Lyme Brain symptoms improve with the ongoing use of teasel root.

I continue to use it because of these clinical findings. However, my research revealed that clear information was not widely available on the extent to which it can cross the blood-brain barrier.

OLIVE LEAF EXTRACT

Olive leaf extract is well known for its immune-boosting properties and antioxidant properties. It is antibacterial, antiviral and antifungal, and has been used extensively to keep gut flora in balance, guarding against Candida overgrowth and Helicobacter pylori (an infection of the stomach that reduces our ability to produce stomach acid and, hence, digest proteins). It has strong antiviral activity, too, and as many Lyme patients are cross-infected with viruses, this is a valuable trait. I have recently added olive leaf extract to my Lyme Support Formula to provide all these benefits.

Historically, olive leaf extract has been used to treat malaria, demonstrating its efficacy against parasites and its usefulness in Babesia treatment. In fact, I remember a patient with Lyme and Babesia who I treated a few years ago. She was getting ready to start treatment when her husband got a transfer to Japan. Rather than try to negotiate treatment and manage antibiotics abroad, she opted to defer her treatment for six months. Instead, she started on olive leaf extract and built up to relatively high doses. Six months later, she returned to the U.S. symptom free from Babesia!

I have done trials with olive leaf since, and while not everyone is going to get that degree of benefit, I have seen it make a significant contribution to Babesia and Lyme treatment.

Olive leaf's active ingredient is oleuropein. Different products have different levels of this constituent, and higher levels will provide greater benefit. Oleuropein has beneficial effects on blood pressure and cardiovascular function, too.

Of most significance for those with Lyme Brain, research demonstrates that olive leaf extract protects the brain from damage caused by degenerative diseases such as Alzheimer's and Parkinson's disease. It does this through its anti-inflammatory and antioxidant actions.

One study found that in the animals that were pretreated with olive leaf extract and then subjected to a medically induced stroke, there was a marked decrease in damage to brain tissue and a 55% reduction in the volume of dying brain tissue as compared to the control animals.[2] In chronic degenerative illness, olive leaf can help prevent neurofibrillary tangles that can result from inflammation and the accumulation of abnormal proteins in the brain, tangles that can grossly impact cognitive function and memory.

Olive leaf has also been shown to reduce the permeability of the blood-brain barrier. As we know, chronic infections such as Lyme can release toxins and promote inflammation in the body; if the blood-brain barrier is "leaky," more of those toxins can cross into the brain and cause neurological issues. The only advantage of this would be that more antibiotics could cross over into the central nervous system, but there are many disadvantages. What causes a "leaky" blood-brain barrier? Severe infections and the inflammatory changes they produce, for one. Remember how we discussed in the first section that severe acute infections such as meningitis can cause leakiness of the blood-brain barrier? There is also some evidence that gluten can promote greater permeability, too—just another reason to stay away from it! But we'll talk more about that later in the Nutrition section.

Overall, olive leaf extract is not considered one of our prime Lyme fighters because there are herbs that are more effective against the spirochetes themselves. I do think, however, that given its other properties, it is definitely worth considering in treatment protocols, especially in those with known parasitic and viral elements.

ARTEMISININ

Another herbal antimicrobial that is commonly used in Lyme treatment is artemisinin. It is an extract from the herb Artemesia annua, or sweet wormwood. Artemisinin is most commonly used to address Babesia, as it has strong antiparasitic properties. Historically, it has been used extensively to treat malaria, which has many similarities to Babesiosis.

Interestingly, not all Artemesia contains artemisinin, which is why I always recommend that my patients take the extract itself, not just the whole herb. There are also other derivatives of artemisinin. Artemether (employed by the pharmaceutical industry—the medication Coartem [aka Riamet] contains a combination of artemether and lumefantrine, for example) is fat-soluble, can cross the blood-brain barrier and has a long life span in the body, but it is also the most toxic form. Artesunate is another derivative. It is water soluble and highly active but has a very short life span in the body. Artemisinin is the safest choice of those that cross the blood-brain barrier and has a decent life span in the body.

Artemisinin also has anti-inflammatory properties. It is thought to promote healthy NF-kappa Beta levels. This is a molecule in our bodies that detects threats to cells, such as toxins and infectious agents and, subsequently, turns on the genes that promote inflammation. With unchecked NF-kappa Beta, inflammation is perpetuated, contributing further to chronic disease.

CRYPTOLEPIS SANGUINOLENTA

Cryptolepis has a long history of use in African countries to treat malaria. Research shows that the active constituent, indoquinoline alkaloids, has activity against the Plasmodium species, the parasites that cause malaria.[3,4]

Because Babesia is a malaria-like illness, there will be similarities in treatments, and we can draw from centuries of traditional medicine use for our remedies. Hence, today, cryptolepis is used for Babesia treatment in the realm of tick-borne illness.

Once again, information on whether cryptolepis crosses the blood-brain is limited. I could find some opinions but nothing really solid. I include it here because I do have patients who Herx on cryptolepis, and part of that Herx can be brain-related symptoms. That would suggest that it is getting some blood-brain barrier penetration.

HOUTTUYNIA CORDATA

Houttuynia is an herb that has demonstrated activity against Bartonella, a common co-infection of Lyme. I have found that Bartonella can cause a lot of neurological symptoms; in fact, it is a hallmark of Bartonella that neurological symptoms are out of proportion to musculoskeletal symptoms. I have several patients who have said to me, "My body is fine. It's my head that's a mess," and those patients often have Bartonella as their dominant infection. Other than symptoms similar to Lyme Brain (e.g., cognitive issues, memory loss and trouble with focus), Bartonella tends to create more severe anxiety, panic attacks, obsessive-compulsive traits and so on. I do see all of these flare up in some patients when Houttuynia is commenced (for some, at very low doses).

Houttuynia is one of my go-to herbs for Bartonella, and I use it extensively. Once again, solid information on blood-brain barrier penetration is scarce, but given its ability to cause such severe neurological Herxes and subsequent improvements, Houttuynia is certainly impacting the brain-related symptoms.

This is just a sampling of the many antimicrobial herbs that are used in the treatment of Lyme and its co-infections. For some, there is clear information on which ones cross the blood-brain barrier and, for others, trying to find that information was like searching for a needle in a haystack! Therefore, in severe cases of Lyme Brain, it seems logical to lean more towards the ones with clear research and information that support their penetration of the blood-brain barrier.

Herbs that do cross the blood-brain barrier:

- ❖ Garlic

- ❖ Andrographis

- ❖ Japanese Knotweed

- ❖ Cat's Claw

- ❖ Olive Leaf Extract

- ❖ Artemisinin

Herbs with uncertain blood-brain barrier penetration:

- ❖ Teasel Root

- ❖ Cryptolepis

- ❖ Houttuynia

REFERENCES

[1] Buhner, Stephen Harrod. *Healing Lyme: Natural Healing and Prevention of Lyme Borreliosis and Its Coinfections.* San Diego: Raven Press, 2005.

[2] Mohagheghi, F, M R Bigdeli, B Rasoulian, P Hashemi, and M R Pour. "The neuroprotective effect of olive leaf extract is related to improved blood-brain barrier permeability and brain edema in rat with experimental focal cerebral ischemia." *Phytomedicine*, January 2011: 18(2-3):170-5.

[3] Cimanga, K, T De Bruyne, L Pieters, A J Vlietinck, and C A Turger. "In vitro and in vivo antiplasmodial activity of cryptolepine and related alkaloids from Cryptolepis sanguinolenta." *J Nat Prod* 60 (1997): 688-691.

[4] Kirby, G C, A Paine, D C Warhurst, B K Noamesi, and J D Phillipson. "In vitro and in vivo antimalarial activity of cryptolepine, a plant-derived indoloquinoline." *Phytother Res* 9 (1995): 359-363.

CHAPTER 13
ANTI-INFLAMMATORIES

———◇◇◇———

CURCUMIN

Curcumin, a constituent of turmeric, has been used for centuries as an anti-inflammatory and antioxidant agent. It is also used in autoimmune issues to regulate immune function. There are many studies demonstrating its efficacy in reducing inflammation and the mechanisms by which it reduces inflammation. One such mechanism is reducing pro inflammatory cytokines such as IL-1, IL-6, COX2, MMP-9, NF-kB, CRP and TNF, many of the same cytokines that are found to be elevated in Lyme patients. As an antioxidant, curcumin increases levels of vitamins C and E, and prevents lipid peroxidation and oxidative damage.[1]

Curcumin also reduces oxidative damage caused by D-galactose, a reducing sugar that can cause mitochondrial dysfunction and apoptosis (death) of neurons. A study demonstrated that D-galactose did indeed cause cognitive deficits, biochemical changes and demonstrable changes in the tissues. Curcumin effectively reduced oxidized lipids, and improved mitochondrial enzymes and glutathione levels. A summary of the study concluded that "curcumin and hesperidin protect morphological facets and improve biochemical functions of neurons thereby improving cognition."[2]

Equally beneficial for Lyme Brain is evidence that curcumin can help regenerate and repair cells in the brain. Research shows that a component of turmeric known as aromatic-turmerone can increase neural stem cell growth in the brain by up to 80%.[3] Neural stem cells differentiate into various types of neurons—nice, new, healthy neurons! The study found that the number of actual stem cells produced increased with exposure to curcumin, and also that the stem cells increased the number of fully differentiated neural cells.

Other research shows that curcumin can help prevent the accumulation of beta-amyloid plaques in the brain, the very plaques that are found in Alzheimer's disease and other degenerative neurological conditions.

Curcumin may also be protective against various toxic metals such as copper[4] and aluminum.[5] Certainly, toxic metals are common in Lyme patients and can significantly contribute to Lyme Brain.

Curcumin can enhance DHA levels in the brain.[6] DHA is one of the vital fatty acids that support brain health, and deficiencies have been linked to several cognitive disorders, including anxiety. DHA is either obtained through the diet or created from dietary precursors; however, the conversion rate is low. Curcumin increases the conversion of the precursor alpha-linolenic acid to DHA. It also increases levels of the enzymes needed to synthesize DNA, such as FADS2 and elongase 2, in both the liver and brain tissues. Given that many people avoid seafood due to concerns about mercury toxicity, a deficiency of DHA may be a contributing factor to Lyme Brain. Curcumin can help the body to produce more DHA from other dietary sources.

Curcumin is a very safe and non-toxic substance with a good track record of success. Studies have shown effective doses to be as low as 150mg to 500mg.[7] There have been over 60 clinical trials on the safety and efficacy of curcumin in humans and another 35 trials evaluating its efficacy. As with many substances found in nature, curcumin has multiple benefits: regulating the immune system, reducing inflammation, acting as a neuroprotective agent and promoting neural regeneration. Curcumin C3 Complex as well as liposomal curcumin formulations show promising results.

BOSWELLIA SERRATA

Boswellia is a plant that is often used as an herbal extract. I will include it in our discussion on essential oils for brain function, but due to its common use as an herbal medicine, I'll touch on it here, too.

Boswellia has a long history of use in arthritis and arthritic conditions. Research demonstrates both a reduction in pain and an improvement in function when compared with a placebo.[8, 9] It is said to inhibit a pro-inflammatory enzyme known as 5-lipoxygenase and has been used in place of NSAIDs, in many cases with great results. 5-lipoxygenase generates inflammatory leukotrienes, which cause inflammation by promoting free radical damage, cell adhesion and the migration of inflammation-producing cells to the inflamed area. It has also been used in inflammatory bowel conditions, such as Crohn's disease, and respiratory issues such as asthma, partially through the inhibition of 5-lipoxygenase but also via inhibition of the pro-inflammatory enzyme human leukocyte elastase.

Another use for Boswellia is to regulate cell proliferation, or curb the unhealthy division and reproduction of cells, in cancer. It has been shown to inhibit glioblastomas, a type of tumor in the brain, as well as other cancers.[10,11] It is also used to reduce brain edema associated with chemotherapy and radiation therapy in cancer treatment.[12]

In fact, research shows benefit for edema secondary not only to cancer but also to chronic inflammatory diseases. Since inflammation and edema in the central nervous system are one of the known mechanisms of Lyme Brain, Boswellia shows promising application here.

While Boswellia is well known for its anti-inflammatory benefits for arthritis and musculoskeletal pain, it also shows good promise for helping the general inflammation that can contribute to Lyme Brain. As an added benefit, it has fewer gastrointestinal side effects because it works by reducing 5-lipoxygenase and not by inhibiting COX-2 as NSAIDs do. The problem with NSAIDs is that they also block the COX-1 enzyme that is needed to maintain a healthy stomach lining. With prolonged use, over-inhibition of these enzymes can render the stomach lining susceptible to damage.

Having said all of that, I tend to use Boswellia more in the form of the essential oil Frankincense, but more on that later!

STEPHANIA ROOT

Stephania root is a potent anti-inflammatory, in particular, modulating NF-kappa Beta and IL-6, two pro-inflammatory cytokines frequently elevated in Lyme patients.[13] Those inflammatory cytokines can contribute to microglial activation, resulting in neurological symptomatology. The constituent of stephania called tetandrine (TET) is one that has been documented in the medical literature to be the most effective. The tetandrine works to reduce microgial activation via reduction of nitric oxide and superoxide anion generation in the brain.

Stephania crosses the blood-brain barrier, making it ideal for Lyme Brain-related symptoms. There are two primary kinds of stephania found in herbal tinctures and supplements—Stephania tetrandra and Stephania cepharantha. According to Stephen Buhner, they work equally well. Logically enough, the tetandrine constituent is primarily found in S. tetrandra.

Stephania helps with cognitive function and also the promotion of a healthy memory. It has been used to reduce Bell's palsy and trigeminal neuralgia, both which involve cranial nerves.

One of stephania's active ingredients, (-)-stepholidine (SPD), helps to balance the dopaminergic pathways in the brain, improving the linkage between D1 and D2 receptors. This is one of the ways that stephania helps Lyme Brain, but it also reduces the motor symptoms of Parkinson's disease (when administered with levodopa, also called L-dopa) and improves schizophrenic behavior.[14]

SDP has neuroprotective activity, functions as an antioxidant and slows neuronal degeneration in a part of the brain called the substantia nigra.

The aforementioned TET also appears to be neuroprotective and has been shown to reduce neurological injury, including after ischemic strokes. One study demonstrated that TET given post-infarct reduced neurological deficits, the size of the area of damage and also brain edema.[15] While I recognize that Lyme disease and strokes are different issues, it is important to recognize the value of this compound in neurological healing and protection, which is applicable regardless of pathology.

Another study showed benefit in refractory epilepsy, partially by reducing the seizure rate overall and partially by potentiating anti-epilepsy drugs in this population (patients with refractory epilepsy are resistant to anti-epileptic drugs).[16] This may also benefit some Lyme patients who experience seizures and/or seizure-like activity through enhancing the stability of the neurological system.

PROTEOLYTIC ENZYMES

Many people are familiar with enzymes as something you take with your food to help you digest it better. But there is another form of enzyme that is taken away from meals on an empty stomach, for the purpose of breaking down some of the inflammatory debris that is created within the body. I think of them like Pac-Man in the body. They chomp through the inflammatory muck, helping to reduce pain and swelling. Proteolytic enzymes can help reduce the swelling of tissues, decrease capillary permeability, and dissolve clots and tissue deposits.

Proteolytic enzymes include bromelain, papain, pancreatin, trypsin, chymotrypsin, and rutin. They function to help support immune function in a number of ways, including their ability to break down antigen-antibody complexes and increase the capability of macrophages and natural killer cells.

Proteolytic enzymes also reduce fibrin, which is a fibrous mesh that forms around cells in areas of tissue damage. This can be lifesaving, as this is the mechanism for forming a blood clot in acute injury, but studies show an association between chronic ongoing fibrin activation, and chronic disease and inflammation.

Too much fibrin impedes the flow of blood and results in hypercoagulation. Many Lyme patients seem to have elevated fibrin and subsequent "sticky blood." This can impede healthy circulation and oxygenation of the tissues, compromising the flow of nutrients into the cells and waste products out of the cells. It can also compromise the ability of therapies, such as antibiotics, to reach areas of infection.

Another important aspect of this is that fibrin can form a kind of scaffolding from which biofilm can hang and prosper. Biofilm is "sticky goo" (yes, that's a scientific term!) that is created by bacterial colonies and serves as a hiding place for them. We know that addressing biofilm is crucial in Lyme treatment in order to allow antimicrobial therapy to penetrate tissues and seek out all the pathogens.

Proteolytic enzymes have also been shown to be involved in the catabolism of peptide neurotransmitters and structural proteins in the brain; hence, they can assist with healthy neurological function and may help in cases of depression and anxiety.

As with many of the anti-inflammatories, proteolytic enzymes are not used specifically for brain function, but by virtue of supporting immune function, reducing inflammation and breaking down biofilm to enhance activity of antimicrobials, they can have positive results for patients with Lyme Brain.

They are usually taken in capsule form and, importantly, on an empty stomach. We are not looking to digest our food better in this context; therefore, taking them away from food is imperative.

REFERENCES

[1] Rai, Balwant, Jasdeep Kaur, Reinhilde Jacobs, and Jaipaul Singh. "Curcumin exhibits anti-pre-cancer activity by increasing levels of vitamin C and E, and preventing lipid peroxidation and oxidative damage." *J Oral Sci* 52, no. 2 (2010): 251-6.

[2] Banji, Othila J F, David Banji, and Kalpana Ch. "Curcumin and hesperidin improve cognition by suppressing mitochondrial dysfunction and apoptosis induced by D-galactose in rat brain." *Food Chem Toxicol* 74 (2014): 51-9.

[3] Hucklenbroich, Joerg, et al. "Aromatic-turmerone induces neural stem cell proliferation in vitro and in vivo." *Stem Cell Res Ther* 5, no. 4 (September 2014): 100.

[4] Wan, Xiao-hua, Yu-wen Li, and Xiao-ping Luo. "Curcumin attenuated the lipid peroxidation and apoptotic liver injury in copper-overloaded rats." *Zhonghua Er Ke Za Zhi* 45, no. 8 (August 2007): 604-8.

[5] Sood, P K, U Nahar, and B Nehru. "Curcumin attenuates aluminum-induced oxidative stress and mitochondrial duysfunction in rat brain." *Neurotox Res* 20, no. 4 (2011): 351-61.

[6] Wu, A, E E Noble, E Tyagi, Z Ying, Y Zhuang, and F Gomez-Pinilla. "Curcumin boosts DHA in the brain: Implications for the prevention of anxiety disorders." *Biochim Biophys Acta* 1852, no. 5 (May 2015): 951-61.

[7] Aggarwal, Bharat B, Subash C Gupta, and Bokyung Sung. "Curcumin: an orally bioavailable blocker of TNF and other pro-inflammatory biomarkers." *Br J Pharmacol* 169-8 (2013): 1672-1692.

[8] Cameron, M, and S Chrubasik. "Oral herbal therapies for treating osteoarthritis." *Cochrane Summaries*, May 2014.

[9] Kimmatkar, N, V Thawani, L Hingorani, and R Khiyani. "Efficacy and tolerability of Boswellia serrata extract in treatment of osteoarthritis of knee-randomized double blind placebo controlled trial." *Phytomedicine* 10, no. 1 (January 2003): 3-7.

[10] Winking, M, S Sarikaya, S Rahmanian, A Jodicke, and D K Boker. "Boswellic acids inhibit glioma growth: a new treatment option?" *J Neurooncol* 46 (2000): 97-103.

[11] Park, Y S, J H Lee, J Bondar, J A Harwalkar, H Safayhi, and M Golubic. "Cytotoxic action of acetyl-11-keto-beta-boswellic acid (AKBA) on meningioma cells." *Planta Med* 68, no. 5 (2002): 397-401.

[12] Weber, C C, K Reising, W E Muller, M Schubert-Zsilavecz, and M Abdel-Tawab. "Modulation of PGP Function by Boswellic Acids." 72, no. 6 (May 2006): 507-13.

[13] Xue, Y, Y Wang, D C Feng, B G Xiao, and L Y Xu. "Tetrandrine suppresses lipopolysaccharide-induced microglial activation by inhibiting NF-kappaB pathway." *Acta Pharmacol Sin* 29, no. 2 (February 2008): 245-51.

[14] Yang, K, G Jin, and J Wu. "The neuropharmacology of (-)-stepholidine and its potential applications." *Curr Neuropharmacol* 5, no. 4 (December 2007): 289-94.

[15] Ruan, L, H S Huang, W X Jin, H M Chen, X J Li, and Q J Gong. "Tetrandrine attenuated cerebral ischemia/reperfusion injury and induced differential proteomic changes in a MCAO mice model using 2-D DIGE." *Neurochem Res* 38, no. 9 (September 2013): 1871-9.

[16] Chen, Y, X Xiao, C Wang, H Jiang, Z Hong, and G Xu. "Beneficial effect of tetrandrine on refractory epilepsy via suppressing P-glycoprotein." *Int J Neurosci* 125, no. 9 (2015): 703-10.

CHAPTER 14

DETOXIFICATION SUPPORT

GLUTATHIONE

Anyone who knows me knows that I'm a huge fan of glutathione. Among its many other benefits, I have seen it help with Lyme Brain in so many of my patients.

Two of glutathione's primary roles are to act as an antioxidant and neuroprotector, and to facilitate detoxification. Thirdly, and less well known, is glutathione's ability to support neurotransmitter levels and, hence, mood. Glutathione is one of the most important substances I know of to keep the brain healthy and functioning well.

Glutathione is one of the brain's most significant protectors, functioning as its master antioxidant. While the brain only accounts for 2% of body weight, it consumes 20% of the body's oxygen. Therefore, the brain produces a high proportion of reactive oxygen species. Glutathione is one of the key defenses to counter these reactive oxygen species, which can otherwise be quite damaging because they produce oxidative stress and neuronal cell damage.

Low glutathione has been associated with Alzheimer's disease and Parkinson's disease. Amyloid-B peptide is one of the substances that have been implicated in plaque accumulation in Alzheimer's disease, resulting in neurological degeneration. Glutathione has been shown to prevent the death of brain cells induced by amyloid plaques.[1] Research also shows that in Alzheimer's patients, high homocysteine levels correlate with low cognitive performance and low glutathione levels.[2]

In addition to being the key antioxidant for the brain, glutathione plays a significant role in detoxification by combining with toxic elements and allowing their excretion from the body. Deficiencies in glutathione impair our ability to detoxify harmful substances. Conversely, the toxic substances themselves can deplete glutathione, so it's a double-edged sword.

There are many toxic insults to the brain—e.g., toxic metals, mycotoxins and pesticides—and all can, and do, deplete glutathione. Poor diet, stress, trauma, chronic infections, aging, medications and radiation can further deplete glutathione. And yet, glutathione is key to detoxing these toxic agents and countering these biological stressors.

There are also genetic factors that can lead to the reduced production of glutathione. This is certainly one of the reasons why some people have such a high toxic load and an impaired ability to clear them from the body. This "glutathione crisis" occurs in many chronic illnesses and is seen extensively in Lyme patients.

I do have some people who do not tolerate glutathione well. Those with extreme sulfur sensitivity may not do well with it, as it is a sulfur-based compound. Certain methylation defects will also make one less tolerant of glutathione, but in my clinical experience, this is the minority. Most people need glutathione, and even if they have a detoxification response in the early phases of treatment with it (thus requiring low starting doses and a gradual build up), they ultimately benefit from it. Many patients have told me that their cognitive function has improved immediately upon starting glutathione. I know for myself, if I have a long day with patients or a period of writing where I need to focus, I'll take a shot of glutathione first!

The third and less well-recognized benefit of glutathione is in balancing brain chemistry. In fact, studies have shown significant improvements in social behavior in cases of depression and bipolar disorder with supplementation of N-acetyl cysteine (NAC), a precursor to glutathione.[3]

It is thought that glutathione makes receptors in the brain more sensitive to dopamine and serotonin, two crucial neurotransmitters for healthy brain function. Further, antidepressants have been found to deplete glutathione, again setting up yet another double-edged sword: the medications taken to help depression may worsen one of the contributing factors to the depression itself.

You can see now the importance of healthy glutathione levels. In our population of Lyme patients, with their high levels of inflammation in the brain often coupled with infection in the brain and a myriad of other exogenous toxins, there are frequently depleted glutathione levels. And yet, these are exactly the circumstances that create a high requirement for glutathione.

One of the issues in boosting glutathione is how to effectively supplement it. Many oral supplements of glutathione are not effective, as they break down in the digestive tract and cannot be well absorbed and utilized by the body. Liposomal glutathione is an exception to this and the form that I use extensively. The way that liposomal glutathione is created allows it to be absorbed across the mucous membranes of the digestive tract without being "digested" and broken down in the gut. Intravenous glutathione is also a great form, but for many people can be harder to access.

Some people prefer to supplement with the precursors to glutathione, most notably N-acetyl cysteine (NAC). I still prefer the liposomal glutathione directly, as I have found NAC to promote Candida issues in some patients. Curcumin can also boost glutathione levels, adding to its lengthy list of benefits; however, I do not rely on it alone to support glutathione. Undenatured whey protein is another way to boost intracellular glutathione. I'm not a big fan of dairy, so although a pure whey protein doesn't contain casein, which is the more problematic component of dairy, and might have certain benefits, I still advise against its use in many of my patients. Liposomal glutathione is my first choice because it is so effective.

SMILAX GLABRAE

Smilax glabrae is one of my favorite herbs in Lyme treatment, especially for Lyme Brain. Smilax glabrae does cross the blood-brain barrier and is used to help neutralize neurotoxins. It also has anti-inflammatory properties, which add to its benefit.

Smilax has a long history in treatment protocols for syphilis, which is also a spirochetal bacterial infection.

Michael Murray, in *The Healing Power of Herbs* writes:

> *"French physician Nicholas Monardes described its use in 1574 to treat syphilis. Since it was assumed that Christopher Columbus's crew had brought the syphilis epidemic in Europe from the Americas, it was felt that the cure might lie in America's herbs. A study done by the British of Portuguese soldiers in 1812 showed that the soldiers suffering from syphilis who were treated with sarsaparilla recovered much faster than those treated with mercury (the treatment of choice in those days). The Chinese also used sarsaparilla to treat syphilis, and through blood tests, showed that sarsaparilla was effective in 90% of cases of acute syphilis and 50% of cases of chronic syphilis."[4]*

While it's not my herb of choice for actually addressing the microbial aspect of Lyme, it has huge value in Lyme Brain due to its ability to cross the blood-brain barrier. The glabrae form of Smilax is the form with the best blood-brain barrier penetration. I have not seen other forms have the same benefit, so the glabrae form of the herb is very important here.

Smilax glabrae is helpful for offsetting Herxheimer reactions in 90% of my patients. In some of my highly sensitive patients, I have seen it cause some Herx or detox reactions. Therefore, there is a wide range of dosing of this herb. Some people start with 1 drop a day, while others can go straight to 30 drops of the tincture twice daily. For the most sensitive individuals, I have had them place 1 drop in one liter of water and take 2–3 sips per day for the first few days.

Along with working directly in the brain, Smilax also has the ability to neutralize endotoxins in the intestines. Many endotoxins are cleansed from the gut by the lymphatic system and liver. Binding the toxins in the gut before they reach the bloodstream helps to minimize the inflammatory response they can cause.

Another potential role of Smilax glabrae is to provide protection against the harmful effects of toxic metals. One study evaluated the effects of lead acetate on oxidative stress in the brain and found that Smilax glabrae showed significant efficiency in reducing blood and tissue levels of lead.[5] It also increased protective antioxidants such as superoxide dismutase and the ever-important glutathione.

Given that many Lyme patients struggle with heavy metals, and toxic metals can contribute to Lyme Brain, this added benefit makes Smilax a great option.

In addition to detoxification support, Smilax glabrae has known anti-inflammatory properties. Studies show that two of the key constituents, SGP-1 and SGP-2 (both polysaccharides) are responsible for this action and suppress the release of nitric oxide, tumor necrosis factor-alpha, and interleukin-6—all mediators of inflammation that are elevated in Lyme patients.[6]

Certainly the benefit my patients get from Smilax for their body pain further supports this research on Smilax's anti-inflammatory action.

I find that Smilax combined with glutathione is my winning combination for supporting Lyme Brain. Together, they typically have a huge impact, more than any other herbs or supplements I have found. I would add the essential oil Frankincense to complete the trifecta!

PIMPINELLA ANISUM

Pimpinella has the ability to cleanse toxins, both endogenous (created by the body itself) and exogenous (taken in from external sources), from the nervous system. It has been used to slow neurodegeneration and may also have the ability to cleanse heavy metals from the neurological system.

Pinella is a product that is used extensively in the Cowden protocol as a "Brain/Nerve Cleanse." It is an extract from the Peruvian herb Pimpinella anisum. It is frequently coupled with Burbur, which also supports detox, but Pimpinella has the stronger affinity for the central nervous system.

One study at the University of Guayaquil in Ecuador demonstrated that the product Pinella inhibited inflammation by 51.2%.[7] Knowing that inflammation is a chief cause of Lyme Brain, this result is significant. Pimpinella is also very safe, has no known contraindications, and has low toxicity and side effect profiles.

Another manifestation of Pimpinella anisum is anise. Anise comes from the seeds of the plant, while some pimpinella herb extracts comes from the bark. Anise can be taken in tincture form or, in some cases, used as an essential oil. I have less experience with anise for Lyme Brain, and there is limited information published on it. In a study on the use of anise oil in seizure disorders and hypoxia of the brain (low oxygen status), anise reduced the frequency of seizure activity and reduced its severity. It also showed benefit in cases of hypoxia, demonstrating a neuroprotective effect.[8]

With some promising preliminary research, and the fact that it is derived from the same plant as the Pimpinella extract which can cross the blood-brain barrier, it may be useful for some people to combat Lyme Brain.

MOLYBDENUM

Molybdenum is a trace mineral that can play a significant role in detoxification. I believe that it is not utilized frequently enough, but I have seen it be hugely beneficial to my patients, especially those who have major issues with Candida.

One way it works is to assist the detoxification of acetylaldehydes. Acetylaldehydes are part of the larger aldehyde family, which are environmental toxins. Sources include alcohol consumption, cigarette smoke, smog, industrial pollution and synthetic fragrances. Most notably for Lyme patients, acetylaldehydes are released by Candida albicans, so those with an overgrowth of Candida likely have elevated acetylaldehydes. Since these can accumulate in various tissues, including the brain, it follows that acetylaldehyde toxicity contributes to their Lyme Brain.

If acetylaldehyde is a waste product of Candida, then we need to address both the Candida itself as well as the toxic byproducts. Molybdenum is a safe and effective way to promote the breakdown of acetyladehyde. By breaking it down to acetic acid, the body has a better chance of eliminating it. The body can also convert acetic acid to acetyl coenzyme A, which is part of the body's energy production system. Molybdenum along with iron and thiamine is needed for the enzyme reactions that underpin that conversion.

One symptom that I have observed in my patients is waking up in the early hours of the morning. Candida is a major cause of that. Anecdotally, I have seen cases where a dose of molybdenum in the middle of the night (through its action of breaking down the acetyladehydes that can cause the night waking) will help people get back to sleep.

As a side note, perfumes and fragrances today contain mostly toxic chemicals—up to 90% petroleum-based—rather than natural scents. Many of those toxic chemicals are aldehydes. Therefore, a Lyme patient (or any individual) who already has Candida overgrowth as one source of aldehydes is more likely to be tipped over the edge by synthetic fragrances, another source of aldehydes. Molybdenum can help in these cases to reduce the brain fog and other associated neurological symptoms.

There are two other benefits of molybdenum worth noting. Firstly, molybdenum and zinc help to keep copper levels in check by competing with copper for similar absorption sites in the gut. If copper levels are too high in the body, it can act as a toxin, similar to lead or mercury. Therefore, if laboratory testing shows high copper in relation to zinc, supplementing with both zinc and molybdenum will help bring it back in balance. The second benefit is that low molybdenum levels are correlated with high sulfites, which can lead to sulfite sensitivity and allergy. Just as molybdenum is a component of the enzyme aldehyde oxidase, it is also part of sulfite oxidase. Molybdenum can help people become more tolerant of sulfites.

YUCCA

Yucca extract comes from the desert plant Yucca schidigera. It is frequently used to assist in the detoxification of ammonia in the body and brain.

One of the potential sources of Lyme Brain is elevated ammonia levels in the body. This may be due to certain methylation defects, which can lower BH4 and impact one's ability to detoxify ammonia. David Jernigan describes the release of ammonia as a byproduct of the Borrelia bacteria itself and views ammonia as one of the major endotoxins in Lyme patients.[9] Ammonia accumulation in the brain can subsequently be a factor in Lyme Brain, in particular, through its impact on neurotransmitter receptors and altered brain energy metabolism.

Patients with high levels of ammonia should also watch their protein intake because protein digestion and metabolism naturally produce ammonia. Most of us have adequate systems for breaking down proteins without accumulating unhealthy levels of ammonia, but if the liver detoxification systems are not functioning adequately, ammonia levels may build up. Or, if methylation and other genetic factors predispose one to high ammonia, it may be worth considering reducing one's protein intake.

Interestingly, Yucca has also demonstrated anti-inflammatory effects. It contains phenolic compounds, which inhibit NF-kappa Beta, ultimately leading to higher levels of nitric oxide and lower levels of inflammation in the body. The same phenolics have been shown to be free radical scavengers that suppress reactive oxygen species.[10]

Yucca is not my first choice of a detoxification aid, unless I have a patient with known elevations in ammonia levels. In those cases, though, it can be a great aid to detox substances that can contribute to toxicity and Lyme Brain.

REFERENCES

[1] Lee, Jiunn-Tay, Jan Xu, Jin-Moo Lee, and Grace Ku. "Amyloid- peptide induces oligodendrocyte death by activating the neutral sphingomyelinase–ceramide pathway." *J Cell Biol* 164, no. 1 (January 2004): 123-131.

[2] McCaddon, A, et al. "Alzheimer's disease and total plasma aminothiols." *Biol Psychiatry* 53, no. 3 (February 2003): 254-60.

[3] Dean, Olivia, Frank Giorlando, and Michael Berk. "N-Acetlycysteine in psychiatry: current therapeutic evidence and potentialmechanisms of action." *J Psychiatry Neurosci*, March 2011: 78-86.

[4] Murray, Michael T. *The Healing Power of Herbs: The Enlightened Person's Guide to the Wonders of Medicinal Plants.* 2nd. Rocklin: Prima Publishing, 1995.

[5] Xia, D, X Yu, S Liao, Q Shao, H Mou, and W Ma. "Protective effect of Smilax glabra extract against lead-induced oxidative stress in rats." *J Ethnopharmacol* 130, no. 2 (July 2010): 414-20.

[6] Chuan-Li, L, et al. "Polysaccharides from Smilax glabrae inhibit the pro-inflammatory mediators via ERK1/2 and JNK pathways in LPS-induced RAW264.7 cells." *Carbohydr Polym* 122 (May 2015): 428-436.

[7] Nutramedix: Bionatus Laboratories. "Pinella: Brain/Nerve Cleanse." *Bionatus Nutramedix News and Research.* http://www.nutramedix.ec/pdfs/Pinella_flyer.pdf (accessed 2015).

[8] Karimzadeh, F, et al. "Anticonvulsant and neuroprotective effects of Pimpinella anisum in rat brain." *BMC Complement Altern Med* 12, no. 76 (June 2012): 76.

[9] Jernigan, David. "Lyme-Induced Leaky Brain Syndrome." *Dr. David Jernigan, Hansa Center: Advanced Alternative Healthcare for Chronic Illness. Changing Lives, Not Just Bodies.*™. http://davidjernigan.blogspot.com/search?q=ammonia+ (accessed 2015).

[10] Cheeke, P R, S Piacente, and W Oleszek. "Anti-inflammatory and anti-arthritic effects of yucca schidigera: A review." *J Inflamm (Lond)* 3 (2006): 6.

CHAPTER 15

NEUROTRANSMITTER SUPPORT

$$\longrightarrow \diamond \bowtie \diamond \longrightarrow$$

As we learned in Section 1, one of the contributing factors to Lyme Brain is an imbalance in neurotransmitters. If you recall, neurotransmitters are chemicals in the brain that assist in nerve conduction from one nerve to the next. They are released at the end of the nerve fiber with each nerve impulse, and then they are carried with the nerve impulse on to the next cell. Imbalances in neurotransmitters can cause major issues such as anxiety, depression, issues with memory, cognition and mental processing—all the things we usually associate with Lyme Brain.

Many Lyme patients have neurotransmitter imbalances; in general, many people have neurotransmitter imbalances. If you consider the size of the pharmaceutical industry, specifically antidepressant and anti-anxiety medications, the scope of the problem becomes clear. Those medications are a multibillion-dollar industry.

Any neurological illness can deplete neurotransmitters. Methylation defects also impact neurotransmitter production and utilization. Because many Lyme patients experience methylation gene mutations, it makes sense that so many have issues with neurotransmitter balance. Neurological illness creates a higher need and demand for neurotransmitters, so there is the double-edged sword of increased need with depleted supply.

There are four major ways to manipulate neurotransmitter levels: 1) Selective re-uptake inhibitors increase their levels in the synapse of neurons by preventing them from being reabsorbed back into the neuron they were expelled from; 2) receptor agonists enhance the effects of neurotransmitters on receptor binding sites; 3) neurotransmitter substrates increase the amount of neurotransmitters produced; and 4) enzyme modulators influence the actions of specific enzymes that influence neurotransmitter levels. Pharmaceutical companies aim to create medications that influence one or more of these factors.

One of the challenges with that is that in many cases, the limiting factor is not enough of the neurotransmitter to start with. Let's take the case of selective serotonin reuptake inhibitors. They function by preventing the reuptake of serotonin back into the neuron, thus lengthening its action as a messenger between cells. But what if there are low levels of serotonin to start with? All the recycling in the world can't correct fundamentally low levels, even though they can successfully prolong and optimize the activity of what is there.

One of the modalities that I find so helpful in Lyme patients, especially for helping Lyme Brain, is amino acid therapy. Amino acid therapy is a way to naturally and safely increase the supply of the raw materials the body needs to produce neurotransmitters. We can supplement with the building blocks so that the body can take those raw materials and create more neurotransmitters. The raw materials are specific amino acids that fuel specific neurotransmitter pathways. This often brings relief from many psychoemotional symptoms, without the many side effects of prescription antidepressants.

People who are already on antidepressant or anti-anxiety medications can also benefit from amino acids therapy, but it must be done under the supervision of a physician to make sure levels remain in balance. Serotonin syndrome occurs when levels of serotonin get too high, so if one is taking SSRIs, for example, it would not be wise to take large doses of 5-HTP. I highly recommend Julia Ross's book *The Mood Cure* for very detailed information on amino acid therapy for pain, mood and other neurological issues.

Each neurotransmitter has its own pathway and uses different amino acids. Three of the major pathways are the serotonin pathway, the dopamine/norepinephrine pathway and the GABA pathway. I have included a simplified representation of those pathways.

SEROTONIN

Tryptophan => 5-hydroxytryptophan => serotonin =>
5-hydroxyindoleacetylaldehyde (5-HTP) => n-acetylserotonin
=> Melatonin

NOREPINEPHRINE

Phenylalanine => Tyrosine => L-Dopa => dopamine => norepinephrine
=> epinephrine

GABA

Glutamine => Glutamate => GABA

SEROTONIN PATHWAY

You can see that the serotonin pathway starts with tryptophan and moves through 5-HTP to become serotonin. Interestingly, serotonin is converted to melatonin, so people with chronic insomnia can also benefit from supporting the serotonin pathway.

Many people associate tryptophan with the post-turkey dinner sedative effect! That, in its most basic form, is an example of an amino acid fueling a neurotransmitter pathway and, in this case, creating more serotonin and melatonin. Of course, that might not be ideal for anyone's productivity, so people turn to supplements for a more regulated and metered dose (without the extra calories of all the turkey trimmings!).

Once upon a time, tryptophan was used extensively as a supplement in the United States. Sadly, due to a contamination issue, it was restricted by the FDA in 1989 and got some bad press around that time. Today, tryptophan can be found in supplemental form, but 5-HTP has taken over in popularity. In other countries, tryptophan is widely available.

5-HTP, or 5-hydroxytryptophan, is the molecule that is made from tryptophan and goes on to become serotonin. Supplementing with 5-HTP gives the body the raw materials it needs to produce its own serotonin and melatonin. For these reasons, it can have tremendous benefit in depression and in anxiety, too. Serotonin is an inhibitory neurotransmitter (i.e., it has a calming effect on the brain). 5-HTP tends to be calming and balancing, and relieves depression. In larger doses, it can help push the pathway towards melatonin and assist in sleep.

I usually prefer GABA over 5-HTP for anxiety, but for some people, 5-HTP is more effective. As with so many elements of Lyme treatment, it is worth trying one at a time and seeing which one causes a better response.

EPINEPHRINE PATHWAY

The epinephrine pathway uses the amino acid phenylalanine, which moves through tyrosine to become dopamine, norepinephrine and epinephrine. Most people are familiar with Parkinson's medications, which work by increasing dopamine to stabilize neurological function.

I use tyrosine more extensively than phenylalanine to support this pathway. In her book *The Mood Cure*, Julia Ross talks about using phenylalanine to relieve pain as well as depression, fatigue and cravings. The d-form of phenylalanine is better for pain relief, while l-phenylalanine is more stimulating (and logically, the dl-form is a combination of both).

Tyrosine in supplemental form is helpful for depression with extensive fatigue, low moods, apathy, low libido, poor concentration and focus. I choose tyrosine when "the blahs" seem to be dominant in the depression picture and 5-HTP when anxiety and feeling wired occur with it. Some people do well with both, but of course, I recommend starting one at a time.

Tyrosine also functions to support the thyroid, so in some cases, supplementing can boost energy and metabolism through optimizing thyroid function. Those taking thyroid hormone medication and/or other thyroid boosters (e.g., glandulars and iodine) should monitor their thyroid levels when starting to take tyrosine.

I have also used tyrosine in cases of inattentiveness, lack of focus and memory loss—all the cognitive elements we observe in Lyme Brain. Julia Ross uses it to assist in addiction recovery with excellent results.

Too much tyrosine can be too stimulating, so it is wise to start slowly and build incrementally.

GLUTAMINE-GABA PATHWAY

The GABA pathway starts with glutamine. However, in this particular case, we actually supplement with GABA itself rather than the precursor glutamine. One reason for this is that it is available in supplement form as actual GABA, so it does not even require any processing or synthesizing by the body. Also, while glutamine is an amino acid that can have some benefit in the brain, high glutamate is excitatory and causes more problems than it solves. Therefore, to avoid the risk of too much glutamate actually opposing the desired result, which is a calmer brain, we supplement with GABA itself. Supplemental GABA is also the antidote to high glutamate.

I have found GABA to be very helpful for anxiety. Some of my patients have been able to get off benzodiazepines with the use of supplemental GABA, as it provided enough of the calming effect they needed without the risk of dependence and withdrawal concerns. I have found a derivative of GABA called Phenibut (4-amino-3-phenylbutyric acid) that seems even more effective than plain GABA. My favorite product containing this derivative is called Phenitropic by Biotics.

THE NEUROTRANSMITTER ACETYLCHOLINE

Acetylcholine is another neurotransmitter that is found in the central nervous system. It is associated with memory and learning, and is a target for therapies and medications to slow the progression of Alzheimer's disease.

Its synthesis requires choline, acetyl CoA (a product of cellular metabolism) and the enzyme choline acetyltransferase (amongst other things, but that's the simplified version).

Acetylcholine is also tied into methylation pathways too, as you can see in the following diagram:[1]

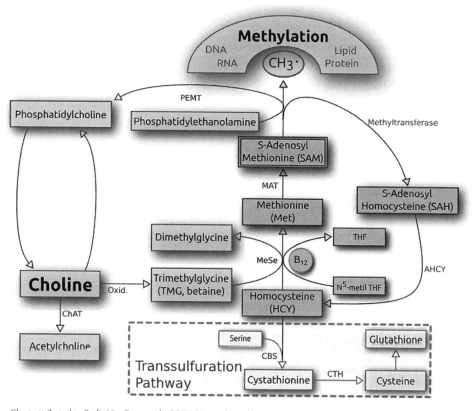

Chart attributed to Radio89 - Own work, CC BY-SA 3.0, https://commons.wikimedia.org/w/index.php?curid=20265140

It is thought that the typical diet is quite deficient in choline. Eggs are a good source, as is lecithin (so these two things might be helpful for people who are depleted). Other sources are beef liver, lean beef, chicken and wheat germ. According to the National Health and Nutrition Examination Survey in 2003, only 10% of the population gets adequate choline.[2] That means that 90% of the population may be deficient in choline. This may explain why people are impacted by problems with acetylcholine production and are wandering around with poor memories and cognitive function. Neurons cannot synthesize choline; it must be obtained from the diet.

Studies show that high choline levels correlate with lower levels of anxiety. No association was found between choline status and depression rates.[3]

As it relates to Lyme disease, it has been proposed that Lyme disease patients have lower acetylcholine due to a blockage in production by toxins released by the Borrelia bacteria.[4] Certainly the cognitive elements of low acetylcholine fit with the cognitive symptoms of Lyme Brain.

From a supplement standpoint, lecithin is perhaps the most readily available source of choline. However, simply increasing choline in the brain does not necessarily increase acetylcholine synthesis; other precursors and conditions must exist. Because acetylcholine needs choline plus an acetyl group, we frequently see acetyl-L-carnitine being given to provide that acetyl group. Phosphatidylcholine can be used to contribute to choline status and can be taken orally or via IV. Phosphatidylcholine has benefits in supporting membrane integrity and mitochondrial function, which can help with the chronic fatigue that many people experience.

Phosphatidylserine is another molecule that can be taken supplementally to support acetylcholine. Studies have found that phosphatidylserine enhances the supply and utilization of acetylcholine in the brain. It also appears to increase brain turnover of dopamine, norepinephrine and glucose.

For these reasons, phosphatidylserine has been reported to enhance brain function, memory, cognition and mood, and reduce anxiety and relieve depression. A study at the University of Milan showed that in women suffering from depression, phosphatidylserine reduced depression and anxiety, and improved long-term memory and learning.[5] Another study showed that phosphatidylserine may help brain metabolism. After just three weeks of supplementation, PET scans showed enhanced cellular activity in all regions of the subject's brain.[6]

Further research is needed to fully understand other ways to support acetylcholine production. This will probably be an area that has application in Lyme treatment and will benefit those with Lyme Brain. For now, adding supplemental lecithin along with acetyl-L-carnitine and/or phosphatidylserine appears to provide the best combination.

※

Generally speaking, amino acid therapy is a very safe way to support Lyme Brain recovery. It can lead to a more balanced and even mood, less depression and anxiety, better focus and concentration, and even things like less cravings, increased libido, and lower pain levels. As I mentioned, for those already taking pharmaceutical medications that influence neurotransmitter levels, greater care must be taken to keep everything in balance, and physician supervision is recommended. Clinics such as the Amen clinic and Julia Ross's clinic (The Nutritional Therapy Institute Clinic) provide assistance to patients in this capacity also.

Of all the interventions for Lyme Brain that I discuss in this book, amino acid therapy is at the top of my list of most helpful therapies. I have seen it give many people great help and support for emotional and cognitive balance. It is an inexpensive, safe and widely available tool.

REFERENCES

[1] Anonymous. "Choline." *Wikipedia: The Free Encylopedia.* 2016   17-March. https://en.wikipedia.org/wiki/Choline.

[2] Zeisel, S H, and Kerry-Ann da Costa. "Choline: An Essential Nutrient for Public Health." *Nutr Rev* 67, no. 11 (November 2009): 615-23.

[3] Bjelland, Ingvar, Grethe S Tell, Stein E Vollset, Svetlana Konstantinova, and Per M Ueland. "Choline in anxiety and depression: Tthe Hordaland Health Study." *Am J Clin Nutr* 90, no. 4 (October 2009): 1056-1060.

[4] Bradford, Robert W, and Henry W Allen. "Biochemistry of Lyme Disease: Borrelia Burgdorferi Spirochete/Cyst." *Townsend Letter, the Examiner of Alternative Medicine.* 2006   February/March.

[5] Maggioni, M, et al. "Effects of Phosphatidylserine Therapy in Geriatric Patients With Depressive Disorders." *Acta Psychiatr Scand* 81 (1990): 265-270.

[6] Klinkhammer, P, B Szelies, and W D Heiss. "Fffect of phosphatidylscrine on cerebral glucose metabolism in Alzheimer's disease. Dementia." *Dementia* 1, no. 4 (1990): 197-201.

CHAPTER 16

COGNITIVE SUPPORTS/ NEUROPROTECTIVES/ANTIOXIDANTS

—=><=—

VINPOCETINE

Vinpocetine is an extract from the plant lesser periwinkle (Vinca minor). It has a long history in Europe as a remedy for cognitive decline, stroke recovery and epilepsy.

One of vinpocetine's primary benefits is to increase blood flow and, hence, oxygenation to the brain. It inhibits the enzyme phosphodiesterase type 1 (PDE1), which normally causes smooth muscle contraction and reduces intracellular calcium, resulting in constriction of blood vessels and reduced blood flow through the vessels. Relaxation of the smooth vessels allows greater blood flow. Greater blood flow means more oxygen and nutrients can be delivered to brain cells, and more carbon dioxide and waste products can be removed from the brain cells. Inhibition of PDE-1 also has antioxidant benefits, resulting in less stickiness of the blood and platelet clumping. It can minimize damage to nerve cells in cases where there is limited blood supply.

Vinpocetine has been demonstrated to increase glucose supply and metabolism in the brain. Glucose is the brain's primary source of fuel, so a brain that doesn't have sufficient glucose will not function optimally. This effect was proven via PET imaging in Hungarian studies.[1,2]

It increases mitochondrial function, too, which further increases energy production. It is also neuroprotective and capable of reducing neural inflammation and hyperexcitability. It curbs inflammation by inhibiting tumor necrosis factor-alpha

(TNF-α)-induced NF-κB activities. This is of major significance to Lyme patients where chronic inflammation is so common.

As an antioxidant, vinpocetine demonstrates hydroxyl radical scavenging properties and reduces intracellular reactive oxygen species. This means it can contribute to the reduction of toxins and other harmful molecules that can damage brain cells and compromise cognitive function. It has reduced seizure activity by suppressing neuronal hyperexcitability.

Vinpocetine easily crosses the blood-brain barrier. From examining the research, it appears that the most promising mechanism by which vinpocetine can assist with Lyme Brain is through the increase in blood, glucose and oxygen flow. Neuroprotective, antioxidant and anti-inflammatory effects are a secondary bonus!

HUPERZINE A

Huperzine A is a naturally occurring compound extracted from Chinese club moss Huperzia serrata (also found in lower proportions in other species of Huperzia). Its main mechanism of action is as an acetylcholinesterase inhibitor, which means it stops the enzyme acetylcholinesterase from breaking down acetylcholine, with the net result being greater bioavailability of acetylcholine. As we now know, higher acetylcholine levels have been associated with enhanced cognitive function.

Huperzine A has been examined for some time as a potential treatment for Alzheimer's and other degenerative neurological diseases. A secondary effect of huperzine A is that it reduces neurotoxicity by interfering with beta-amyloid deposition in the brain, which is one of the major sources of neurodegeneration, particularly in Alzheimer's.

Many studies and animal models have demonstrated the benefits of Huperzine A. A study in China found benefit in elderly people with benign senescent forgetfulness (aka "normal" memory loss associated with old age, not caused by a specific disease).[3] Another one, also in China, found benefit to school age children reporting memory decline.[4]

I have found that Huperzine A does make a difference in cognitive function in Lyme patients. Although anything that increases acetylcholine can have cholinergic side effects, including nausea, vomiting, blurred vision, restlessness, sweating and reduced heart rate, I have found Huperzine A to be safe and non-toxic in recommended doses.

LITHIUM

When we hear about lithium and neurological health, we often think of the pharmaceutical form of lithium, which is primarily used in bipolar disorder. There is also what we term nutritional lithium. It is a different form given in much lower doses, typically doses of 5mg to 20mg in the orotate form, while the drug Lithium (in carbonate form) can be given up to 2000mg daily.

Lithium orotate is an over-the-counter supplement, and I have seen it work very well in stabilizing mood and promoting healthy psychoemotional states. Technically, lithium is a trace mineral, so supplementing with it is no more extreme than supplementing with potassium, magnesium or iodine. All are minerals and all can benefit the body if naturally occurring levels are depleted. The orotate form has excellent blood-brain barrier penetration, and its high bioavailability is purportedly one of the main reasons it can be so effective at such modest doses.

One study from Texas of 27 state counties between 1978 and 1987 found that the counties that did not have lithium in the water had much higher rates of violent crime (such as murder and rape), suicide and drug addiction. In fact, the counties whose water contained lithium had 50% lower rates in all these variables.[5]

"Harvard Medical School has analyzed over 30 human meta-analysis studies and has determined that lithium reduces the rate and risk of suicide attempts by 80-90% in patients with major depression, bipolar disorder, and schizoaffective disorder. The overall risk of suicide was five times lower among lithium-treated subjects compared with individuals not treated with lithium."[6]

Lithium can act as a neuroprotectant, reducing excessive levels of various neurotransmitters that might be excitatory (such as the glutamate that we discussed in the last section or excesses of norepinephrine and epinephrine that can become too stimulating to the brain). It can also stimulate neurogenesis (production of new neurons). It stimulates stem cells in the hippocampus of the brain to prevent the loss of proliferation induced by high glutamate or high cortisol. Longer-term treatment with lithium then promoted the conversion of the stem cells into neurons.[7]

Lithium, as well as reducing excess glutamate and norepinephrine, also supports and boosts serotonin, which is one of the key mechanisms by which it helps depression. It can also protect the brain from exogenous toxins such as heavy metals and reduces arachidonic acid in the brain, a fatty acid that contributes to inflammation. Many people have found relief from headaches and migraines using lithium orotate. Improvements in cognitive function are typical. This occurs via its ability to support healthy brain receptor function and brain signaling cascades, along with the balancing of neurotransmitters.

Lithium at such low doses (5mg to 20mg) seems to be extremely safe and very few side effects are reported. I have had a few patients get a bit zoned out/spacey if they took a dose that was too high for them. For depression, headaches/

migraines, memory loss, cognitive dysfunction and post-traumatic stress disorder, lithium orotate is an inexpensive and safe supplement to trial.

VITAMIN B12

When we think of B12, we often think of its energy-boosting properties, and it certainly has those, but what is less well known about B12 is its profound impact on and benefit for the brain. This is a double bonus for Lyme patients who have chronic fatigue *and* Lyme Brain.

B12 deficiency is widespread. Results from the Framington study indicate that of the 3,000 men and women studied, 39% registered in the low-normal range—below 258 picomoles per liter. A diagnosis of B12 deficiency requires levels below 148 pmol/L, and there were only 9% that met that criterion. However, since many people will exhibit neurological limitations at low-normal levels and not just "deficient" levels, this diagnostic criterion can be tricky and may miss many situations where B12 therapy could help neurological and cognitive health.[8] Again, testing methylmalonic acid may be a better indicator, but my advice most of the time is just to supplement with B12 and see if it helps (with the type of B12 given determined by methylation testing). Another factor to remember is that B12 taken orally is not well absorbed. B12 given by injection (or IV) is the best form for absorption, and sublingual is a decent runner-up.

One of the important factors is the role of B12 in methylation. B12 is often supplemented in the form of methyl-B12. The methyl groups in that compound can provide methyl donors to fuel the methylation cycle. Much like an engine of a car, without the right fuel and adequate oil and water, the engine cannot perform optimally. While a detailed discussion of methylation is beyond the scope of this book, it is important to understand that one of the things the methylation pathway does is regulate neurotransmitter production. We have already learned how impactful that can be for emotional regulation as well as learning, cognition and memory. Methylation also drives detoxification. Individuals with toxic assault on their brain from neurotoxins, heavy metals, mold toxins and so on can benefit from supporting methylation (even though the detox effect can be rugged in the beginning). I have certainly found in my Lyme patient population that the majority of people are undermethylators and, therefore, benefit from methyl-B12 as well as other methylated forms of B vitamins such as 5-methyl-tetrahydrafolate. Some people, though, are overmethylators, and for them, the methyl-B12 might make things worse. They might need a different form such as hydroxy-B12.

Other than its role in methylation, B12 also has several benefits for the brain. It has been found to improve blood-brain barrier function in people with cognitive impairment. By measuring proteins in the central nervous system, it was determined in one study that B12 (along with folate and B6) tightened the junctions of the blood-brain barrier; a lower percentage of protein was detected in the cerebro-spinal fluid after 270 days on the nutrient supplements.[9] Cognitive function was also stabilized in these patients. This demonstrates that good cognitive function is compromised when blood-brain barrier strength is compromised, which occurs when there is chronic inflammation in the body and brain.

Other research indicates that a B12 deficiency can lead to brain shrinkage (yikes!).[10] This study was published in the Neurology journal and demonstrated some interesting points. The first is that serum B12 itself is not a good indicator of B12 status, rather B12 markers such as methylmalonic acid and homocysteine should be examined. Lower B12 status markers correlated not only with total brain volume, but with global cognitive function. This is why B12 deficiency in the aging population is associated with high rates of dementia and cognitive decline, and possibly also Alzheimer's disease.

Vitamin B12 is also needed to produce the protective lining around nerves known as the myelin sheath. Demyelination of that sheath occurs in diseases such as multiple sclerosis and other degenerative neurological conditions. Given that the myelin sheath is involved in nerve impulse signals traveling from one nerve to an-other, it follows that if that structure is weak, nerve signaling will be compromised. This can manifest as memory loss, difficulty with focus/concentration, word-find-ing difficulties and slurred speech.

Interestingly, a study that looked at MRI imaging of people with B12 deficiency and neurological symptomatology demonstrated that B12 deficiency does indeed present with focal demyelination of white matter in the spine and optic nerve and, in some cases, presents with a white matter pattern typically seen in multiple sclerosis patients.[11]

Many a Lyme patient has had a brain MRI, and many have demonstrated white lesions. In most cases, this has prompted discussions with neurologists about MS, and often a di-agnosis of MS was made. We know that Lyme disease can produce white matter lesions on MRIs, and B12 deficiency should be considered as an additional or alternative cause.

RESERATROL

We talked about the herb Polygonum cuspidatum in the section on antimicrobial treatments for Lyme Brain. Here, I want to specifically discuss resveratrol, a poly-phenol compound. Polygonum (or Japanese knotweed) is a source of resveratrol, but there are other sources including red wine, red grapes, dark chocolate, pea-nuts and mulberry skins.

Resveratrol is touted as an anti-aging supplement and has also been used to support brain and cognitive function. Certainly, resveratrol acts to increase circulation in the brain, and the increase in blood flow can bring more oxygen into the cells and remove wastes from the cells. It has strong antioxidant properties, which led to its popularity as an anti-aging supplement, but it also has the ability to activate a family of proteins called sirtuins, which have been connected to longer age span, lower incidence of cancer, enhanced metabolism and overall better health.

Until recently, human studies demonstrating the benefits of resveratrol on brain function were somewhat limited, although animal studies always supported the hypothesis. Old mice given resveratrol supplements every day performed better on spatial learning and working memory tests than non-supplemented mice.[12]

More recently, a German research group sought to determine if resveratrol did indeed improve cognition, brain function and memory in humans.[13] They gave 23 adult participants 200mg of resveratrol daily for 26 weeks, while 23 controls took a placebo. The results showed that the resveratrol boosted the participants' ability to recall words; it increased the functionality of the hippocampus, the area of the brain involved with formation, organization and storage of memory; and it reduced glycated hemoglobin (HbA1c), demonstrating that it helps to regulate blood sugar, which can also protect the neurological system. This study does support the role of resveratrol, not only in general wellbeing and anti-aging, but also as a valuable supplement for cognitive function.

ACETYL-L-CARNITINE

Acetyl-L-carnitine was mentioned briefly in the section on acetylcholine support as a possible donor of the acetyl group required to make that particular neurotransmitter.

Even outside of that role, acetyl-L-carnitine has long been used for brain and cognitive support, and there is much research supporting its use and benefit. It is way more absorbable than regular L-carnitine, and the acetyl-L form has superior blood-brain barrier penetration, which is desirable for those needing help with Lyme Brain.

There are several mechanisms by which acetyl-L-carnitine helps the brain. It is a nutrient that helps to produce energy, thus fueling the cells, boosting their metabolism and making them function better. It does this by reducing glucose metabolism to lactate.[14] It also helps to metabolize fat and cholesterol so that the brain does not get clogged with plaques and deposits.

Acetyl-L-carnitine can help to prevent the buildup of amyloid plaque, which can contribute to cognitive decline. It does this by promoting the production in nerve cells of alpha-secretase instead of beta-secretase, resulting in less beta amyloid plaque. It boosts levels of brain-derived neurotrophic factor (BDNF), which helps to repair damaged cells and even produce new brain cells.

Acetyl-L-carnitine boosts nerve transmission. One study showed that diabetic neuropathy was helped significantly by consistent daily dosing.[15] Patients reported less neuropathic pain, improvement in nerve conduction and some nerve regeneration.

It helps to repair myelin sheaths (as we discussed, B12 can too). While mechanisms are not fully understood, research points to a regulation of the myelin basic protein (MBP) gene, which modulates the turnover of myelin basic protein, thus stabilizing and maintaining membrane integrity.[16]

It also helps to repair any damage to the blood-brain barrier caused by alcohol and other toxins, inflammation etc. It does this by boosting the antioxidant enzymes that naturally protect the blood-brain barrier from toxic stress. Because we know that inflammatory damage to the blood-brain barrier can contribute to cognitive issues, neurological degeneration, reduced learning, memory decline and depression, acetyl-L-carnitine can help to offset such damage and, for this reason alone, is an important nutrient.

As an overall antioxidant, acetyl-L-carnitine is highly neuroprotective, boosting glutathione levels in the brain.

In terms of neurotransmitters, we saw that acetyl-L-carnitine supports acetylcholine. It also has been found to support dopamine levels. Research shows that there is a decline in dopaminergic receptors with age, but that administration of acetyl-L-carnitine for a 3-month period diminished the reduction in binding.[17]

Another study showed that acetyl-L-carnitine increased norepinephrine in the hippocampus and serotonin in the cortex.[18] Supporting norepinephrine and serotonin in the brain can help with depressive symptoms as well as cognitive deficits. This study also confirmed acetyl-L-carnitine's ability to boost brain cell metabolism and energy.

As you can see, acetyl-L-carnitine may be one of the most important nutrients for the brain. It boosts metabolism, acts as a neuroprotectant, helps the integrity of both the blood-brain barrier and the myelin sheaths around nerves and perhaps, most importantly, has the ability to repair already damaged nerve cells and structures, and promote the creation of new, healthy ones.

From a clinical standpoint, it has the ability to boost working memory and retrieval, relieve depression and enhance overall mood, boost concentration and increase mental energy—all things that would be of benefit in Lyme Brain. It is worth trying for 3–6 months, as improvements do not necessarily happen overnight with this nutrient.

ALPHA-LIPOIC ACID

Alpha-lipoic acid is often used in conjunction with acetyl-L-carnitine. Both have antioxidant, neuroprotective and regenerative effects in the brain. Alpha-lipoic acid also improves blood flow, nerve conduction and metabolism in the brain.

Alpha-lipoic acid can easily penetrate the blood-brain barrier. It has been researched in acute issues, such as arsenic poisoning in the brain through to chronic neurodegenerative conditions, such as dementia and Alzheimer's, with benefit in both realms.

Alpha-lipoic acid functions as an antioxidant to the brain, assisting in the recycling of vitamins C and E, and boosting perhaps the most important nutrient: glutathione. While vitamin C is only water-soluble and vitamin E is only lipid-soluble, alpha-lipoic acid is both water- and lipid-soluble, which gives it greater capacity as an antioxidant and a greater ability to benefit all areas of the body.

This allows for greater regeneration of neurological cells and structures as well as protection against inflammation and toxic assaults. Also, alpha-lipoic acid is metabolized both within the cells and in the extracellular space, and in cell membranes, which means it provides protection in all environments. This gives it its powerful benefit in any conditions resulting from oxidative stress in the brain.[19]

Alpha-lipoic acid has been found to repair the blood-brain barrier. We know by now that the blood-brain barrier is impacted by chronic illness, toxic stress and inflammation—all things that occur in Lyme disease. Similar to acetylcholine, by repairing the blood-brain barrier, alpha-lipoic acid helps the brain to function better.

Alpha-lipoic acid has been used to remove heavy metals, such as mercury, arsenic, lead and cadmium, from the brain. One study set up three different situations: 1) alpha-lipoic acid used as a prophylaxis against acute mercury toxicity; 2) alpha-lipoic acid used as a treatment following acute mercury toxicity; and 3) alpha-lipoic acid used as a prophylactic therapy against long-term exposure to mercury. Toxic impact was demonstrated in the toxic group, and the ameliorating effects of alpha-lipoic acid were found in all three groups.[20]

The importance of effective protection against and detoxification of heavy metals in Lyme patients cannot be understated. Toxic metals can create all the same issues as Lyme disease—cognitive decline, mood changes, memory loss, etc. —and so, toxic metals *in addition to* Lyme are a major set up for Lyme Brain.

In a study of traumatic brain injury in mice, which manifested as histological damage (damage to the cells themselves), reductions in glutathione, increases in inflammatory cytokines in the body, increased blood-brain barrier permeability and edema in the brain, alpha-lipoic acid improved every one of these markers.[21] While traumatic brain injury and Lyme Brain are quite distinct and different pathologies, there is overlap in the end result, and hence, it is still useful to examine the research on different impacts on those end results, even if the cause is not the same.

OMEGA-3 FATTY ACIDS

Having long been recognized as a supplement (and food ingredient) with many benefits, omega-3 fatty acids are a good choice for overcoming Lyme Brain, too. Fish oil is perhaps the best known. It is an oil that is high in omega-3 fatty acids, in particular eicosapentaenoic acid (EPA) and docosahexaenoic acid (DHA), both long-chain fatty acids. Other sources of omega-3s are other cold-water fish, shellfish, krill, algae, plant and nut oils, walnuts and flax seeds. Flax seeds are higher in alpha-linolenic acid, which is a short chain fatty acid. While still providing omega-3s and health benefits, they are less potent than the fatty acids found in seafood products.

Fish oils have been used for traumatic brain injury, inflammatory states, age-related cognitive decline, and in chronic degenerative neurological diseases.

One of the key mechanisms of omega-3s is as an anti-inflammatory. The healthy fatty acids are able to convert into anti-inflammatory prostaglandins while at the same time reducing the pro-inflammatory prostaglandins. PG1s are the anti-inflammatory prostaglandins; omega-3s can boost those, and PG2s are pro-inflammatory; omega-3s can reduce those (this is why avoiding saturated fats is important to avoid creating more PG2s, but more of that in the Nutrition section and even more in my book *The Lyme Diet*). PG3s are a mixed bag, but overall they can help balance excess PG2.

Omega-3 fatty acids can also help with brain repair. Essentially, our brain cell membranes are made up of lipids, or fatty acids, which are components of the cell membranes themselves. In fact, 8% of the brains weight is composed of omega-3 fatty acids; they are the building blocks for 100 billion neurons![22,23]

Omega-3s help keep the membranes fluid, stable, and able to keep the right things in and the right things out, which protects the cell and keeps it functioning optimally. Therefore, providing the body with extra healthy lipids can provide the raw material for the body to repair its own cells.

Omega-3s can also prevent brain atrophy. In other words, they can help reduce the loss of brain cells that occurs over time naturally and can be accelerated in chronic disease. One study published in the journal *Neurology* found that in 1,000 older women, those with higher omega-3 levels in their blood had a 0.7 percent higher brain volume based on MRI scans.[24] Higher omega-3 levels were also associated with greater volume in the hippocampus, the part of the brain associated with memory.

There are correlations between low levels of EPA and DHA, and cognitive decline. Another study observed 819 adults: 229 cognitively normal individuals, 397 with mild cognitive impairment and 193 with Alzheimer's disease. They used neuropsychological testing and MRI imaging every six months to assess the progress. Alzheimer's patients were given the Alzheimer's Disease Assessment Scale while the normal cognition subjects were given the Mini-Mental State Examination. Fish oil supplements improved scores in both populations on both neuropsychological testing modalities while the MRIs demonstrated less atrophy in one or more brain regions.[25]

Low levels of EPA and DHA are also associated with higher rates of anxiety, depression, bipolar disorder and even violent/criminal behaviors. They are also correlated with hyperactivity and attention deficit disorders. Thus, omega-3s are a good treatment option for psychoemotional as well as cognitive issues.

While for most adults a combination of EPA and DHA is optimal, some research shows that children have a greater need for DHA for their developing brains. One study of 33 boys between ages 8 and 10 measured both red blood cell levels of DHA and brain activation levels via MRI.[26] Some were given 400mg of DHA, others 1200mg and yet others a placebo. In the group receiving the highest level of DHA, red blood cell levels of DHA increased by 70%! The MRI showed a significant increase in activation in the dorsolateral prefrontal cortex (the area associated with working memory) in the supplemented group. There were also changes in the occipital cortex, which is the visual processing center, and the cerebellar cortex, which plays a role in motor control. This data suggests that DHA would be a beneficial supplement for the developing brains of children.

Another study at Oxford University in England examined 500 children between the ages of seven and nine, looking at their omega-3 fatty acid status.[27] They found that higher levels of omega-3s, especially DHA, were associated with better reading and memory, and fewer behavioral problems among the children. Lower levels of omega-3s were correlated with higher rates of ADHD. The study also reflected that most of the children had sub-optimal levels—2.45%—where the recommendation for preventing heart disease is 8%. This research also supports the importance of supplementing with omega-3 fatty acids in children.

There is ongoing debate about fish oil versus krill oil. One of the major concerns is that toxic substances such as mercury contaminate many fish. Krill, which are smaller creatures and lower on the food chain, have not accumulated as much mercury along the way. Some prefer krill oil because it can reduce the "fish burps" that may come with fish oil supplements. It is also a greater source of the antioxidant astaxanthin, which renders it stable and resistant to oxidation. For me, as long as the fish oil is from a reputable source (see Putting It All Together/Resources at the end) which tests for any contaminants, I am just as happy with the results I see with it, and I use it extensively with my patients.

LION'S MANE MUSHROOM

Lion's mane mushroom, officially called Hericium erinaceus, is a mushroom that grows on trees and logs, and has been used medicinally in Japan for many years. It is not shaped like a traditional mushroom; instead, it has long cascading tendrils that literally resemble the mane of a lion.

Lion's mane is considered a brain tonic, as it appears to increase Nerve Growth Factor, which is needed for the maintenance and regeneration of nerve cells. The active constituents responsible for this are hericenones and erinacines. Erinacines is the more powerful constituent of the two and easily crosses the blood-brain barrier to influence Nerve Growth Factor production in the brain.

About a dozen studies have been conducted since the early 1990s demonstrating the neuro-regenerative properties of lion's mane. In a 2009 study, 30 Japanese patients with mild cognitive impairment were given the dried lion's mane extract 3 times daily for 16 weeks.[28] The results of the study confirmed that the group who took the lion's mane had significantly higher scores on the cognitive function scale than those who took the placebo. However, within a few weeks of stopping the supplement, those scores decreased again. This study suggests that the lion's mane helped cognition significantly while taking it, but that the benefits did not last once it was stopped.

Studies also demonstrate that lion's mane can reduce amyloid plaque deposition in the brain (amyloid plaques are associated with the inflammation of brain tissue, interference with normal nerve signals and nerve degeneration). This second mechanism of action may give it credibility in preventing dementia and Alzheimer's disease. A mouse study showed that when injected with neurotoxic peptides, resulting in the formation of plaques in the brain, the mice lost their ability to memorize a particular maze.[29] Two groups were then formed: one had a regular diet while the other had 5% lion's mane as part of their diet for 23 days. The latter group showed significant improvement on their maze test, reflecting improvements in memory. Those mice also showed another unexpected gain: their curiosity and willingness to explore new and novel objects over familiar ones was enhanced.

Lion's mane also serves to protect and regenerate the myelin sheath, which is important for the healthy functioning of nerves, and for nerve impulses to travel at their optimal speed and with optimal conductivity. Numerous studies confirm this.

One in particular demonstrated both enhancements in the normal development of myelin as well as the stimulation in myelination where degeneration of the myelin sheath had occurred. It showed that myelination in the presence of the mushroom extract occurred earlier and at a higher rate as compared with controls.[30]

Clearly, lion's mane helps with cognition and memory. However, it may help with depression and anxiety, too. A small study of 30 women in Japan did find that the lion's mane extract reduced depression and anxiety in these subjects.[31]

A question from some of my patients when discussing any mushroom products is the relationship with Candida. Granted, there are some people with severe systemic Candida who should avoid any fungus-related foods and products, including lion's mane. However, it is my experience that people who do not have significant Candida issues, provided they are paying attention to their diet (no sugars, low carbs and minimal fruit) and addressing the Candida with antifungal therapy of some kind, can tolerate medicinal mushrooms without any problem. I have had a handful of patients for whom lion's mane has made a significant difference in their cognition, memory and mood. I am excited to have lion's mane as part of my new Brain Support Formula (see section 9 for details).

PROGESTERONE

You might be surprised to see progesterone in a book on brain health. Most people associate progesterone exclusively with female hormones, but it has a myriad of different functions relative to the brain. In fact, one study in the *Frontiers in Neuroendocrinology* journal states:

> *"Emerging data indicate that progesterone has multiple non-reproductive functions in the central nervous system to regulate cognition, mood, inflammation, mitochondrial function, neurogenesis and regeneration, myelination and recovery from traumatic brain injury."*[32]

One of the major mechanisms of these activities is via progesterone's ability to function as a neurosteroid, a naturally occurring steroid that is produced within the body and functions to alter neural excitability. (Remember here that we have many steroid hormones that are natural to the body and that we would be in trouble without. This differs from pharmaceutical steroids, such as prednisone, which are used as immune suppressants and, in most cases, are detrimental to Lyme patients.) Cells in the brain, spinal cord and peripheral nervous system can all synthesize progesterone from cholesterol, and progesterone is able to access the brain and nerves to bind to progesterone receptors in the brain.

Certainly, in pregnancy, rising progesterone levels serve to offer protection to the fetus from neural excitation that could be damaging to his or her fragile nervous system. In a similar fashion, there appears to be a reduction in seizure activity following traumatic brain injury with progesterone supplementation, indicating a similar mechanism of calming neural excitation.

There has been significant research done over time to assess the role of progesterone in recovery from traumatic brain injury. Results have certainly been mixed, but there is significant data to show that progesterone has a neuroprotective effect. In one clinical study known as ProTECT II, 100 patients with moderate to severe traumatic brain injury were assessed.[33] One group was given the standard treatment for traumatic brain injury while the other was given that same treatment plus three days of intravenous progesterone (the dose was sufficient to create levels that were triple those seen at the end of pregnancy). The mortality rate in the conventional treatment was 33%, and the mortality rate in the group who received progesterone was 13%.

One of the major ways progesterone helps after a traumatic brain injury is by reducing edema in the brain. It does this by inhibiting the expression of the genes that trigger cells to release the inflammatory cytokines that lead to the swelling and edema. It also influences water channels in the brain, allowing the outflow and relieving the pressure of excess fluid. It also inhibits programmed cell death (apoptosis) by upregulating the genes that influence it, thus sparing cells that might otherwise be killed off.

Another of the mechanisms of progesterone's neuroprotective and regenerative effects is by promoting myelination. Similar to B12, lion's mane and acetyl-L-carnitine, progesterone can help support healthy myelination of nerves promoting their growth and repair after damage.

While Lyme and traumatic brain injury are not the same pathologies, we can see certain similarities—inflammation, edema, demyelination and so on. As I've mentioned before, sometimes we have to learn from research on other diseases how certain substances, medicines and protocols impact different aspects of the brain and neurological function. Especially because there is precious little research on the impacts of chronic Lyme disease itself, we can learn from other research and gain insights into what can help our Lyme population.

Some generalized studies exist on the effect of progesterone on cognition. One such study demonstrated a correlation between progesterone levels and cognition in post-menopausal women.[34] The researchers looked at the data of 643 healthy post-menopausal women, ranging in age from 41 to 84, who were part of the Early Versus Late Intervention Trial with Estriol (ELITE) study. They conducted neuropsychological tests to assess cognition and memory. No correlation was found between estrogen and cognition, but a correlation was found between progesterone and cognition, with better outcomes on verbal memory tests and global cognition.

Certainly progesterone can be of benefit to women with Lyme, because Lyme causes such hormonal havoc. I see many women benefit from progesterone supplementation—all month long if they are post-menopausal and only in the second half of their cycle if pre-menopausal. This research (which could also be applied to men, who, by the way, also have progesterone, just not as much as women) points to a possible application of progesterone aside from hormonal considerations.

REFERENCES

[1] Szakall, S, et al. "Cerebral effects of a single dose of intravenous vinpocetine in chronic stroke patients: a PET study." *J Neuroimaging* 8, no. 4 (October 1998): 197-204.

[2] Szilágyi G, Nagy Z, Balkay L, Boros I, Emri M, Lehel S, Márián T, Molnár T, Szakáll S, Trón L, Bereczki D, Csiba L, Fekete I, Kerényi L, Galuska L, Varga J, Bönöczk P, Vas A, Gulyás B. "Effects of vinpocetine on the redistribution of cerebral blood flow and glucose metabolism in chronic ischemic stroke patients: a PET study." *J Neurol Sci* 229-230 (March 2005): 275-284.

[3] Wang, R, H Yan, and X C Tang. "Progress in studies of huperzine A, a natural cholinesterase inhibitor from Chinese herbal medicine." *Acta Pharmacol Sin* 27, no. 1 (January 2006): 1-26.

[4] Sun, Q Q, S S Xu, J L Pan, H M Guo, and W Q Cao. "Huperzine-A capsules enhance memory and learning performance in 34 pairs of matched adolescent students." *Zhongguo Yao Li Xue Bao* 20, no. 7 (July 1999): 601-3.

[5] Schrauzer, G N, and K P Shrestha. "Lithium in drinking water and the incidences of crimes, suicides, and arrests related to drug addictions." *Biol Trace Elem Res* 25, no. 2 (May 1990): 105-13.

[6] Leucht, S, W Kissling, and J McGrath. "Lithium for schizophrenia revisited: a systematic review and meta-analysis of randomized controlled trials." *J Clin Psychiatry* 65, no. 2 (Feb 2004): 177-86.

[7] Chiu, Chi-Tso, and De-Maw Chuang. "Neuroprotective action of lithium in disorders of the central nervous system." *Zhong Nan Da Xue Xue Bao Yi Xue Ban* 36, no. 6 (June 2011): 461-476.

[8] McBride, Judy. "B12 Deficiency May Be More Widespread Than Thought." *United States Department of Agriculture Agricultural Research Service*. 2000 2-August. http://www.ars.usda.gov/is/pr/2000/000802.htm.

[9] Lehmann, M, B Regland, K Blennow, and C G Gottfries. "Vitamin B12-B6-folate treatment improves blood-brain barrier function in patients with hyperhomocysteinaemia and mild cognitive impairment." *Dement Geriatr Cogn Disord* 16, no. 3 (2003): 145-50.

[10] Tangney, C C, et al. "Vitamin B12, cognition, and brain MRI measures: a cross-sectional examination." *Neurology* 77, no. 13 (September 2011): 1276-82.

[11] Misra, U K, J Kalita, and A Das. "Vitamin B12 deficiency neurological syndromes: a clinical MRI and electrodiagnostic study." *Electromyogr Clin Neurophysiol* 43 (2003): 57-64.

[12] Kodali, M, V K Parihar, B Hattiangady, B Shuai, and A K Shetty. "Resveratrol prevents age-related memory and mood dysfunction with increased hippocampal neurogenesis and microvasculature, and reduced glial activation." *Sci Rep* 5 (January 2015): 8075.

[13] Witte, A V, L Kerti, D S Margulies, and A Floel. "Effects of resveratrol on memory performance, hippocampal functional connectivity, and glucose metabolism in healthy older adults." *J Neurosci* 34, no. 23 (June 2014): 7862-70.

[14] Smeland, O B, T W Meisingset, K Borges, and U Sonnewald. "Chronic acetyl-L-carnitine alters brain energy metabolism and increases noradrenaline and serotonin content in healthy mice." *Neurochem Int* 61, no. 1 (July 2012): 100-7.

[15] Evans, J D, T F Jacobs, and E W Evans. "Role of acetyl-L-carnitine in the treatment of diabetic peripheral neuropathy." *Ann Pharmacother* 42, no. 11 (November 2008): 1686-91.

[16] Traina, G, G Federighi, M Macchi, R Bernardi, M Durante, and M Brunelle. "Modulation of Myelin Basic Protein Gene Expression by Acetyl-l-Carnitine." *Mol Neurobiol* 44, no. 1 (August 2011): 1-6.

[17] Sershen, H, Jr., L G Harsing, M Banay-Schwartz, A Hashim, M T Ramacci, and A Lajtha. "Effect of acetyl-L-carnitine on the dopaminergic system in aging brain." *J Neurosci Res* 30, no. 3 (November 1991): 555-9.

[18] Smeland, O B, T W Meisingset, K Borges, and U Sonnewald. "Chronic acetyl-L-carnitine alters brain energy metabolism and increases noradrenaline and serotonin content in healthy mice." *Neurochem Int* 61, no. 1 (July 2012): 100-7.

[19] Packer, L, H J Tritschler, and K Wessel. "Neuroprotection by the metabolic antioxidant alpha-lipoic acid." *Free Radic Biol Med* 22, no. 1-2 (1997): 359-78.

[20] Anuradha, B, and P Varalakshmi. "Protective role of DL-alpha-lipoic acid against mercury-induced neural lipid peroxidation." *Pharmacol Res* 39, no. 1 (1999): 67-80.

[21] Toklu, H Z, T Hakan, N Biber, S Solakoğlu S, A V Oğünç, and G Sener. "The protective effect of alpha lipoic acid against traumatic brain injury in rats." *Free Radic Res* 43, no. 7 (2009): 658-67.

[22] O'Brien, J S, and E L Sampson. "Lipid composition of the normal human brain: gray matter, white matter, and myelin." *J Lipid Res* 6, no. 4 (October 1965): 537-44.

[23] Chang, C Y, D S Ke, and J Y Chen. "Essential fatty acids and human brain." *Acta Neurol Taiwan* 18, no. 4 (December 2009): 231-41.

[24] Pottala, J V, K Yaffe, J G Robinson, M A Espeland, R Wallace, and W S Harris. "Higher RBC EPA + DHA corresponds with larger total brain and hippocampal volumes: WHIMS-MRI study." *Neurology* 82, no. 5 (February 2014): 435-42.

[25] Daiello, L A, A Gongvatana, S Dunsiger, R A Cohen, B R Ott, and Alzheimer's Disease Neuroimaging Initiative. "Association of fish oil supplement use with preservation of brain volume and cognitive function." *Alzheimers Dement* 11, no. 2 (February 2015): 226-35.

[26] McNamara, Robert K, et al. "Docosahexaenoic acid supplementation increases prefrontal cortex activation during sustained attention in healthy boys: a placebo-controlled, dose-ranging, functional magnetic resonance imaging study." *Am J Clin Nutr* 91, no. 4 (April 2010): 1060-1067.

[27] Montgomery, P, J R Burton, R P Sewell, T F Spreckelsen, and A J Richardson. "Low Blood Long Chain Omega-3 Fatty Acids in UK Children Are Associated with Poor Cognitive Performance and Behavior: A Cross-Sectional Analysis from the DOLAB Study." *PLoS ONE* 8, no. 6 (2013): e66697.

[28] Mori, K, S Inatomi, K Ouchi, Y Azumi, and T Tuchida. "Improving effects of the mushroom Yamabushitake (Hericium erinaceus) on mild cognitive impairment: a double blinded, placebo controlled clinical trial." *Phytother Res* 23 (2009): 367-372.

[29] Mori, K, Y Obara, T Moriya, S Inatomi, and N Nakahata. "Effects of Hericium erinaceus on amyloid β(25-35) peptide-induced learning and memory deficits in mice." *Biomed Res* 32, no. 1 (2011): 67-72.

[30] Kolotushkina, E V, M G Moldavan, K Y Voronin, and G G Skibo. "The influence of Hericium erinaceus extract on myelination process in vitro." *Fiziol Zh* 49, no. 1 (2003): 38-45.

[31] Nagano, M, et al. "Reduction of depression and anxiety by 4 weeks Hericium erinaceus intake." *Biomed Res* 31, no. 4 (2010): 231-7.

[32] Brinton, R D, et al. "Progesterone receptors: form and function in brain." *Front Neuroendocrinol* 29, no. 2 (May 2008): 313-39.

[33] Wright, D W, et al. "ProTECT: a randomized clinical trial of progesterone for acute traumatic brain injury." *Ann Emerg Med* 49, no. 4 (April 2007): 391-402, 402.e1-2.

[34] Henderson, V W, et al. "Cognition, mood, and physiological concentrations of sex hormones in the early and late menopause." *PNAS* 110, no. 50 (December 2013): 20290-20295.

CHAPTER 17

ESSENTIAL OILS AND BRAIN HEALTH

⇒〇✕〇⇐

Just two years ago, if someone had mentioned essential oils, I would have had visions of a few drops of lavender on the pillowcase to help with sleep. My knowledge did not extend much beyond that. Today, essential oils are one of my favorite modalities for supporting the health of my patients. There are some that are safe to take internally, and I use them for everything from supporting immune function to balancing emotional states, supporting brain function, reducing inflammation and discomfort, increasing energy and supporting detox.

Today, I'll discuss a few of the oils that I utilize to help the brain, but first I want to explain how and why essential oils are so helpful for the brain. Remember our conversation about antibiotics and which ones cross the blood-brain barrier? Two of the limiting factors were molecule size and lipid solubility; the smaller the molecule and the more lipid-soluble, the better the penetration to the brain. Unfortunately, many antibiotics, especially the ones given orally, have poor statistics in this capacity. Essential oils, on the other hand, have great blood-brain barrier penetration. They are small molecules and they are lipids themselves, so they easily cross the lipid-rich cell membranes. Their ability to also get within cells is one of the key features that give them such profound benefit.

Essential oils have similarities to herbs in that they are sourced from plants. They can also be sourced from fruit. The oils are the volatile aromatic compounds from the plant. They are usually steam distilled from the plant, except in the case of citrus fruits, which are cold pressed from the rind. This differs from herbs, which are usually made from the leaf, seed, bark or roots themselves, not the oils. Essential oils are many times more potent than herbs, up to 60 times or even more. I was surprised myself when I learned that one drop of peppermint oil is the equivalent of 27 cups of peppermint tea! If you're looking to calm the digestion or cool the body overall, it would take a lot of tea to have the same effect as one single drop of peppermint oil.

I have used essential oils extensively with my patients to support their health and with good results. To determine which oils will work best, we need to take a quick look at the chemistry of oils and their constituents.

Sesquiterpenes are key constituents that help the brain due to the ease with which they cross the blood-brain barrier. They help to oxygenate the tissues, balance inflammatory response and calm the nervous system. They can support the endocrine system and have analgesic effects. Some oils that are high in sesqueterpenes are cedarwood, frankincense, patchouli, vetiver, ginger, ylang ylang, myrrh, helichrysim, melissa and black pepper.

Two of my favorite oils for supporting healthy brain function are peppermint and frankincense.

Peppermint is stimulating and good for mental alertness. I recommend high quality oils that can be taken internally, so I either have people put a few drops in a capsule and swallow it, or put a drop or two in water and drink it. Some people enjoy a steam inhalation including peppermint and lemon, and for the hard-core…oregano and/or rosemary. Oregano is a very hot, aromatic and pungent oil, so a very small amount goes a long way. Go slow in the beginning! Inhaling the steam still gets the active constituents close to the central nervous system where they can have benefit.

Another way to use peppermint and one that is very popular for occasional head discomfort is to apply it topically on the skull. Instead of applying directly on the temples, however, a better place is on the skull just above the top of the ear; in broad terms, this is where the temporal artery and nerve run through, so it is good to apply it close to that. Plus, putting oils on the temples increases the chance of having them go in the eyes, which does not feel good at all. If that happens with peppermint or any oil, do not rinse it. Instead apply a carrier oil such as coconut oil or olive oil. That will dilute the essential oil, drawing it out and bringing relief quicker than water.

In my view, frankincense is the very best for brain health— again, so long as the highest quality oils are used. Frankincense works best when taken internally. I either have patients put it directly under the tongue, in a capsule to ingest or, in some cases, on the roof of the mouth (preferably towards the back of the mouth on the soft palate). Frankincense can also be applied to the soles of the feet. The soles of the feet are a good entry point for oils as the skin is quite thin, yet the pores are the largest of anywhere on the body, so systemic absorption is rapid and effective. To promote clear thinking, under the tongue or on the roof of the mouth seems to be the most effective.

Patients love frankincense. It helps with brain clarity, focus/concentration and emotional balance. I have many patients who report that their brain is so much clearer since using frankincense. Frankincense is one of those oils that contain sesquiterpenes, constituents that enter the brain and balance the limbic system, hypothalamus and pituitary gland. I have my patients use 3–5 drops 2 times daily.

Ylang ylang is another oil that I find helpful for brain function. It is also a good hormone balancer and sleep aid, so I think of ylang ylang for many of my female patients who have wacky hormones, insomnia, emotional ups and downs, in conjunction with cognitive challenges. Of course, men, too, can use it with good results.

There are plenty of other essential oils that help with emotional balance. Citrus oils such as wild orange can be very uplifting. They are refreshing, cleansing and energizing. They can evaporate quickly, so using them in a diffuser is a good idea to keep a continual stream of aromatic compounds. In fact, peppermint and wild orange together have been shown to be a great combination for supporting beta brain waves, which are the ones needed to support a healthy, alert and focused mental state. Florals, such as rose and jasmine, are also energizing and can help lift one's mood. They are also good when used aromatically in a diffuser.

Some of my personal favorite oils for resilience to stress and calming the nervous system are the woody oils: sandalwood, cedarwood, vetiver and helichrysum, to name a few. They have very warm and earthy aromas, strong base notes that last a long time and have very calming effects. For this reason, they are used in times of anxiousness, high stress and nervous system overdrive. They can also be very helpful for assisting healthy sleep (lavender and cedarwood is my favorite combination for sleep).

Essential oils can be a great addition to a protocol for brain health. If you could choose only one, choose frankincense. Of course, there are many others, including some not covered here. I have just shared a few of my favorites.

A note about the quality of essential oils: There are a wide variety of brands and qualities. Please contact my office for more information on the oils I recommend. I feel very confident and comfortable with people using those oils internally, but beware: not all oils are created equally. Some have additives and others are synthetic, which means that they are man-made. I cannot stress this enough: do not use essential oils internally unless they are of the highest quality, purity and potency, or they could do more harm than good.

If this list seems overwhelming, do not worry. Towards the end of the book, you will find a table summarizing the different herbs and nutrients and their activities as well as a collection of product suggestions that combine these ingredients efficiently.

SECTION 4:

NUTRITION AND LYME BRAIN

CHAPTER 18

INTRODUCTION

———◦✕◦———

It is no secret that diet and nutrition is key for sufferers of Lyme disease. There is a profound difference in outcomes for those who adhere to a strict diet versus those who eat whatever they like. Those who are careful about what they put into their bodies experience lower levels of pain and inflammation, more energy, more even-keeled emotions. And guess what? Less Lyme Brain.

My first book, *The Lyme Diet*, continues to be a popular guide. Most of my patients want to do whatever they can to feel better, and dietary choices are in some ways the simplest changes they can make (note that I said the simplest, not the easiest—for many, following a special diet requires a lot of effort, organization and discipline). I have always said that Lyme disease is one of the most disempowering diseases, largely because of the lack of acceptance of its mere existence, the subsequent lack of research on treatments and solutions, and the odd stigma that seems to accompany it. Making changes in what you put in your mouth can help you regain a sense of control and can be very empowering. Yes, restrictive diets are challenging—but I have seen the benefits time and time again.

I believe that there are certain core principles for using nutrition to help Lyme Brain. These are similar principles to what I shared in *The Lyme Diet*, so my goal here is to help you understand why they're important and how they specifically impact Lyme Brain.

The following is not an exhaustive list of desirable and undesirable foods; it's more of a guide of the major foods that can play a role, for better or for worse.

CHAPTER 19

LEAKY GUT/LEAKY BRAIN

⚬⋈⚬

Most people are familiar with the concept of leaky gut. This occurs when the gap junctions between the cells of the small intestine open up, which allows larger particles than normal to escape into the bloodstream. This can cause an immune reaction because the larger particles are viewed as intruders. Leaky gut can be caused by a number of factors including gluten intolerance and other food sensitivities, intestinal parasites, bacterial imbalance and Candida overgrowth. Essentially, anything that causes inflammation in the gut can contribute to leaky gut.

Did you know that there is increasing evidence of a phenomenon called leaky brain? The premise is much the same. The gap junctions between the cells of the blood-brain barrier open, which allows the passage of undesirable substances into the brain. We have talked quite a bit so far about the protective role of the blood-brain barrier. That protection is crucial. Otherwise, the brain would be vulnerable and potentially exposed to a myriad of things that could be toxic and harmful to it. The goal of the blood-brain barrier is to allow the passage of oxygen, nutrients and fuel *to* the brain, and the removal of carbon dioxide, waste materials and toxins *from* the brain; it keeps chemicals and toxins out. In some cases, that protection works against us, such as when we would like a great penetration of antibiotics into the brain; however, for the most part, we can be grateful for what it provides for us. Remember, in severe inflammatory states such as meningitis, the blood-brain barrier can become very porous, and all of a sudden, all of those oral antibiotics that don't ordinarily work can get in and work quite well. We also know that Lyme is a chronic inflammatory state—although not to the same extent as something like acute meningitis—and that alone can lend itself to some increased permeability of the blood-brain barrier.

There is emerging evidence that a leaky blood-brain barrier contributes to cognitive decline. Certainly, there is damage to the blood-brain barrier in postmortem studies of Alzheimer's patients. A recent study[1] used MRI imaging to evaluate blood-brain barrier permeability. Results demonstrated an age-related decline in the hippocampus, the area that is critical for learning and memory. The breakdown correlated with mild cognitive impairment, damage to pericytes in the blood-brain barrier (per cerebrospinal fluid analysis) and an increased "leakiness" of the blood-brain barrier.

This is all fascinating, but how does it relate to our discussion on nutrition and Lyme Brain? Certain foods (surprise! surprise!) have been touted as major contributors to leaky brain. That brings us to nutrition tip #1.

NUTRITION TIP #1: AVOID GRAINS, ESPECIALLY GLUTEN

Let us start with perhaps the biggest culprit in promoting inflammation in general and, subsequently, creating leaky brain. Gluten, in my opinion, is the most sinister of foods. There is study upon study showing its inflammatory nature and the detriment it causes the human body and mind.

Gluten stimulates zonulin. Zonulin is a substance that regulates the permeability of the lining of the brain and gut through the activation of epidermal growth factor receptors and protease-activated receptors. It is through this mechanism that gluten contributes to leakiness of the blood-brain barrier. To simplify, gluten increases zonulin. Increased zonulin contributes to greater permeability of the blood-brain barrier. Greater permeability of the blood-brain barrier increases the passage of pro-inflammatory cytokines, heavy metals, environmental toxins and other harmful substances into the brain. This then leads to neurological and cognitive dysfunction.

Of course, any food that provokes an IgG response (i.e., food sensitivities or intolerances rather than full-blown food allergies) can trigger the zonulin activation and contribute to leaky gut and leaky brain. Studies clearly show a relationship between food intolerance and depression via leaky gut and the triggering of inflammatory cytokines that come with it.[2]

Leaky gut also promotes toxicity and inflammation systemically by allowing the release of lipopolysaccharides (LPS). Lipopolysaccharides are naturally contained within the bacteria in our gut flora (of which we have hundreds of trillions). As those bacteria die, the contents should be contained within our intestines and excreted through the stool. When the gut is leaky due to gluten or other inflammatory agents, those LPS products can escape into the bloodstream. At that point they become toxic to our system, fueling inflammation and immune reactions.

A search of the literature reflects a wide variety of neurological issues associated with gluten sensitivity: epilepsy, peripheral neuropathy, headaches, migraines, anxiety, depressive and mood disorders, attention-deficit hyperactivity disorders, autism spectrum disorders and schizophrenia.[3]

Just because you do not have gastrointestinal issues when you eat gluten, do not think that you're immune from the brain issues it can trigger. Studies show that gluten can lead to many neurological disorders, including epilepsy, multiple sclerosis, dementia and peripheral neuropathy, even in people with no overt digestive manifestations.[4]

In fact, one study showed that as many as 57% of people with neurologic dysfunction tested positive for anti-gliadin antibodies, indicating gluten sensitivity even in the absence of full-blown celiac disease.[5]

For more information on gluten, grains and their relationship to leaky brain, I recommend Dr. Perlmutter's books *Grain Brain* and *Brain Maker*.

Adopting a gluten-free diet is key for Lyme patients. However, I do caution people about simply replacing their gluten-containing carbs with gluten-free carbs. I believe it is important to avoid the majority of carbohydrates, especially grains. For a variety of reasons, including minimizing Candida overgrowth and keeping blood sugar stable, a high protein, high fat diet seems to be the healthiest choice for Lyme patients. In my patients, I have noted a significant alleviation of their Lyme Brain symptoms when they adopt a grain-free diet.

For more support and information on the logistics of eating gluten free, I would refer you to my first book *The Lyme Diet*. There are also a plethora of books and websites on eating gluten free and a growing number of gluten-free foods available.

NUTRITION TIP #2: AVOID FOOD INTOLERANCES

This tip overlaps somewhat with our previous discussion of gluten. A lot of the mechanisms are similar, but when we talk about food intolerances, we can really be referring to any food, not just gluten or grains. Also, while gluten can trigger an autoimmune process in the body, IgG food sensitivities are not autoimmune per se. Granted they cause immune reactions and fuel inflammation, but they are not autoimmune in the same way that gluten can be.

Let me also clarify the difference between food allergy and food intolerance. In a food allergy, the immune cell involved is an IgE cell. In a full-blown food allergy, the reaction can be quite severe. For example, an anaphylactic reaction is IgE-mediated. Hives, headaches, rashes and milder breathing difficulties are examples of IgE responses. They also occur immediately upon eating the trigger food. For this reason, most people with true food allergies know about them. If you eat a mango and break out in hives, it is pretty clear what's causing the reaction. Therefore, it is quite easy for people to pinpoint their allergens and avoid them entirely.

Food sensitivities, however, involve a different kind of cell, called an IgG cell. These reactions are slower. In fact, they are called Type IV Delayed Hypersensitivity Reactions, and they can take up to 72 hours to manifest. They do not necessarily cause rashes and/or breathing issues and, in fact, don't necessarily cause any digestive upset either. (I have a lot of people tell me that they're not sensitive or intolerant to dairy, for example, because they do not get digestive problems from it, but that does not rule it out as a possibility.) The symptoms can be subtle—general malaise, headaches, lethargy, muscle weakness, and brain fog. Yep, brain fog is one of the main issues people have. This is because immune reactions in the gut still trigger inflammation, which increases cytokine production which can then travel to the brain, cross the blood-brain barrier and cause brain-related issues.

If any food has the potential to cause an intolerance, then how on earth do we know which ones are affecting us? There are two answers to that.

The first involves an elimination diet. This means stripping the diet down to the bare bones, basically removing any potentially sensitive food. In extreme cases, this means lamb and pears only. Other more liberal plans simply call for the removal of common culprits—gluten-containing grains, nuts, dairy, citrus, eggs, corn, soy and, in some cases, nightshades. The 21-day period of elimination gives the immune system a break and a chance to reset. Then foods are reintroduced one-by-one (no more than one every three days) and reactions evaluated. Typically, once the immune system has had a break from the food for a few weeks, it will mount a larger, more noticeable response when it sees that food again, and that sheds light on what foods need to be avoided or eaten on a rotation basis.

The second and less prolonged way is to do an IgG food sensitivity test. This is typically done either through a blood draw or a finger stick. Laboratories can measure immune reactions to many different foods and be very specific with it. Most tests, for example, will differentiate goat dairy from cow dairy, egg whites from egg yolks, and casein from whey (two proteins in dairy products). I find this testing highly valuable and tremendously helpful in fine-tuning the diet to minimize Lyme Brain.

I could give you many examples of my patients' brain fog improving once they removed their own personal food intolerances, which can be quite unpredictable. For some, garlic can trigger an immune reaction, and for others, blueberries can do it. This shows how individualized some of these issues are. One example that stands out in my memory is of a friend who wasn't even a Lyme patient, but I share this story to exemplify how profound these reactions can be.

My friend, Miss R, owned a personal training studio (she is fit, healthy and sharp as a tack). I did food sensitivity testing with her and one of the foods affecting her was sesame. That seemed odd, because it was not something that she ate a lot. Because she was motivated to be in top health, she removed it from her diet. A couple of months later, we were eating sushi for lunch, and she forgot to ask for a roll without sesame seeds. She ate it anyway, thinking it wouldn't be a big deal. However, she was down for the count all afternoon—fatigued, foggy-brained and headachy. Instead of working out, she went home to take a nap. And this was all from a few sesame seeds! If this was the response in a healthy person with no brain fog, imagine the response in a person who has Lyme Brain and had that susceptibility already.

Food sensitivity testing is not expensive, so I would recommend it for everyone.

NUTRITION TIP #3: AVOID DAIRY

To have a conversation about dairy follows nicely from our discussion about food sensitivities, because dairy is one of the primary foods that people test positive for on the IgG test. Dairy is a very inflammatory food, which we know can potentially worsen Lyme Brain. Dairy can impact us in a few ways. It can be an IgG reaction, which means that the immune system is triggered and inflammation ensues. This reactivity can also potentiate leaky gut, which then allows other food molecules to cross over into the bloodstream and trigger the immune system.

Many people are also lactose intolerant, which means that they are lacking in the enzymes needed to digest dairy adequately. The simple solution for this seems to be lactose-free milk. However, that does not overcome the fundamental issue that dairy proteins are quite hard to digest and that dairy is generally inflammatory.

The two main proteins in dairy are casein and whey. Most of the time, the casein is the bigger problem. That is why some people can tolerate whey protein but not whole dairy products. To me, casein is certainly more detrimental to one's health, and so again, there are times when I am fine with someone using a high quality whey protein powder but not eating dairy products.

The final point about dairy is that goat dairy is much easier to digest than cow dairy, because it is closer in structure to human dairy, which of course, we are de-signed to consume (as babies anyway!). I tell my patients that if they really cannot be dairy free, at least stick with goat dairy and not cow dairy.

This is why the IgG food sensitivity test is so helpful. It tests for casein and whey separately, and it separates goat milk from cow milk, which makes it easier to make decisions about just how strict one needs to be with regards to dairy. Dairy products are third on my list (following gluten and sugar) of dietary no-nos. I definitely encourage my patients to avoid them wherever possible and only use goat dairy if any cheating is going to happen!

NUTRITION TIP #4: EAT FERMENTED FOODS (AND, OF COURSE, TAKE PROBIOTICS)

We just learned how gluten could disrupt the normal healthy gut flora. We also saw how gluten can lead to increased permeability of the blood-brain barrier. Neither of these are positive things.

Research also shows that gut flora can have an impact on the blood-brain barrier. In a landmark study in Sweden,[6] it was discovered that mice that were completely devoid of bacteria in their intestines had a leakier blood-brain barrier. When they were given a fecal transplant (gut bacteria from a healthy mouse were implanted into their intestines), the blood-brain barrier started to heal, and there was an increase in tight junction proteins.

Obviously, reducing the source of dysbiosis is important to maintain a healthy gut lining and, subsequently, a healthy blood-brain barrier. Reducing the intake of sugars and carbohydrates, minimizing antibiotics where possible, and other food intolerances are all key contributing factors. Supplementing with prebiotics and probiotics is crucial, especially for those on antibiotics (but in my view, for everyone) as a source of healthy gut flora.

From a dietary perspective, the research on the gut microbiome and its impact on brain function also calls for an increase in foods to support intestinal flora. These are primarily fermented foods. Examples are kimchi, kombucha, fermented vegetables, sauerkraut, kefir, buttermilk and yoghurt.

Given that many Lyme patients restrict dairy in their diet, they have questions about the use of kefir and yoghurt made from cow's milk. I typically allow high-quality fermented dairy products, as the fermentation process makes them easier to assimilate and digest. However, I definitely would opt for goat milk kefir and yoghurt rather than cow milk, as the proteins are closer to human proteins and, therefore, easier for a human to digest. There are also other forms now, such as coconut water kefir, that avoid the issue altogether and are a good choice.

I also worry that many of the commercially available kefirs are high in sugar and low in active cultures. By far, the best option is to make your own, but if that is not possible, choose smaller, locally produced brands such as those available at farmers markets.

NUTRITION TIP #5: AVOID SUGAR

One of the key tips to minimize Lyme Brain is to avoid sugar. There are a few different reasons for this.

A diet high in sugar is going to impact insulin levels and insulin sensitivity. Chronically high-sugar diets contribute to the impairment of the action of insulin on cell receptors and can potentially lead to insulin resistance. Insulin resistance is associated with lower blood perfusion to tissues. This is because one of insulin's roles is to cause blood vessel dilation, which helps the blood circulate to the tissues. This vasodilator function is reduced in insulin-resistant individuals. Less vasodilation means less blood to the cells, therefore, less oxygen and nutrients are delivered, which can then compromise cognitive function. High sugar levels also damage the blood vessels themselves, and this damage to vessels in the brain can contribute to cognitive decline.

These mechanisms have been backed up by research. Tests show that the highest insulin resistance scores correlate with the longest latency time on a learning and memory challenge.[7]

Studies also show that cerebral hypoperfusion is associated with lower cognitive function scores, and with dementia and lower brain volume![8] Yes, the brain will shrink if it's not adequately fed with blood, oxygen and nutrients.

Another large study showed that elevated glucose levels are associated with dementia, even in non-diabetic people.[9] A study was done of 2067 participants—839 men and 1228 women, 232 with diabetes and 1835 without diabetes. Measures included blood glucose levels and glycated hemoglobin levels (HbA1c). When researchers followed up several years later, they found that 524 participants, 450 of which were not diabetic, developed dementia. In this non-diabetic population, elevated blood glucose levels and HbA1c over the past five years correlated with a higher incidence of dementia. It is accepted and well known that diabetes is a risk factor for dementia, but this new data shows that non-diabetics can be affected in the same way, which makes us realize that sugar levels and brain function are closely tied.

It is clear that high glucose and insulin resistance are bad news for brain function, and this is relevant not only for diabetics, but for anyone who maintains a high blood sugar level. Other than the hypoperfusion mechanism, there is also the aspect of glucose and insulin acting as pro-oxidants, which means that they cause oxidative stress in the brain. Glucose can actually react with oxygen causing reactive oxygen species such as superoxides, hydroxyl radicals and hydrogen peroxide. We know already that neurons can be damaged or killed off by oxidative stress and that Lyme and other chronic infections can themselves contribute to oxidative stress. So why fuel the fire further by eating a high-sugar diet?

Another mechanism, and perhaps the most relevant for Lyme patients, is that sugar fuels the growth of Candida albicans, a naturally occurring yeast in the intestines that can become overgrown. Candida overgrowth has many systemic effects, including brain fog, memory loss, depression, anxiety and neurological dysfunction—symptoms that mimic Lyme Brain exactly!

Remember how we said that Candida can produce acetylaldehydes? These acetylaldehydes act in the brain to damage and even kill brain cells. They can damage the lining of your red blood cells, similar to sugars, as discussed previously. They also cause inflammatory reactions. In short, acetylaldehydes act as toxins in the brain and cause brain fog and emotional lability. People who have systemic Candida issues describe it as feeling drunk all the time—fuzzy, foggy, dizzy and not highly functioning. Judgment can be impaired, and memory and focus are definitely impacted.

Research demonstrates that endothelial cells that line the cerebral blood vessels express a protein that binds to Candida albicans, proteins that are not found in endothelial cells in other parts of the body.[10] Hence, we can see that Candida has a direct point of entry into the brain.

Candida overgrowth not only impacts cognition, but it has a great bearing on emotional states, too, such as depression and anxiety. Even more severe psychiatric disorders, including schizophrenia and bipolar depression, have responded to anti-fungal therapy. In many years of working with autism spectrum disorders, I have seen such a close correlation between yeast overgrowth and cognitive and behavioral states in children.

Risk factors for Candida overgrowth include high alcohol consumption, a high-sugar diet, antibiotic use, eating gluten and other inflammatory foods, and untreated parasitic and bacterial infections of the gut, amongst other things. Interestingly, babies' intestinal tracts are colonized with healthy flora during their passage through their mother's vaginal canal. With the high incidence of Cesarean section births today, many infants are missing out on this benefit, which could impact them in the future.

For Lyme patients, the more pressing issue is that many people are taking or have taken long-term and hefty antibiotic regimens. This can definitely cause a predisposition to Candida overgrowth, yet many people have been helped tremendously by these antibiotics. There are times when they are necessary, but we then have to do everything possible to prevent and minimize Candida issues.

Avoiding dietary sugars is one of the primary ways to do this. Taking good quality probiotics and eating fermented foods is another.

I am often asked about quantities and types of sugar. Isn't fruit sugar okay because it's a "healthy" sugar? Well, certainly fruit provides natural sources of fiber, which help slow the absorption of the sugar in it. Fruit also provides vitamins and minerals. However, in avoiding the fueling of Candida, especially for those on antibiotics, it is often necessary to avoid fruits, too, at least for a time. For those not on antibiotics and without significant yeast issues, I usually advise that one to two servings per day of a low glycemic fruit such as blueberries is acceptable. Certainly, for several different reasons as discussed here, refined sugars are a big no-no during treatment and preferably as a life-long health choice.

NUTRITION TIP #6: AVOID EXCITOTOXINS MSG AND ASPARTAME

Monosodium glutamate, or MSG, is a flavor enhancer that is best known as an additive in Chinese food, but in reality it is added to many processed foods. MSG is a salt of the amino acid glutamic acid, but it is the glutamate form as it is used in our foods. Do you remember our discussion of amino acids and amino acid therapy in Section 3 when we talked about the glutamine-GABA pathway? I stated that high glutamate in the brain could actually be excitatory, compromising cognitive function. An antidote to this is supplemental GABA to get the pathway back in balance. Well, MSG is another source of glutamate in the brain, and it can act in destructive ways. Aspartame works in a similar fashion with similar results.

An excitotoxin is a substance that can excite a cell to the point where it becomes damaged or can even die. Given that there are glutamate receptors in the brain, it is clear that eating MSG can overexcite brain cells to the point of death, too. That is not a scenario that anyone would want, let alone someone already struggling with Lyme Brain.

Abnormalities in glutamate receptors have been associated with many neurological diseases including Huntington's chorea, multiple sclerosis, Alzheimer's, epilepsy, behavioral disorders, psychiatric disorders and autism spectrum disorders. MSG and aspartame can also be very damaging to the developing brain in utero and in children.

Why do food producers put MSG in foods? Because it tricks the taste receptors into thinking that the food has more flavor, is more tender and is more enjoyable; therefore, we'll eat more of it. It also costs less to produce, as they do not need to actually produce a higher quality food; they mask poor quality food with MSG to make it seem better quality. Also, MSG triggers the pancreas to produce insulin, which causes blood sugar to drop and makes us feel hungry again an hour later.

The producers of MSG are aware, of course, that their product has a bad reputation, so in order to circumvent the decline in its use, they change the way it's labeled. Here is a list of foods that can contain MSG:

- ❖ yeast extract
- ❖ autolyzed yeast
- ❖ modified food starch
- ❖ textured vegetable protein
- ❖ hydrolyzed soy protein
- ❖ soy concentrate or isolate
- ❖ natural flavor broth

Some personal care products, such as skin care and hair care products as well as many sunscreens and insect repellants, may also contain MSG.

As for aspartame, the mechanism is similar. It acts as an excitotoxin, damaging the brain cells and potentially killing them. It can also be converted to glutamate and bind with the same receptors that MSG can bind with.

From a dietary standpoint, one of the easiest ways to avoid exposure to MSG and aspartame is to eat whole, unprocessed foods. A diet rich in vegetables, healthy fats and lean proteins will naturally not contain MSG (although some foods have naturally occurring glutamate, such as soy sauce, parmesan cheese, walnuts, peas, seaweed and mushrooms). Once you start eating out a lot, especially at Asian restaurants, and buying packaged/convenience foods, then you're more suscepti-ble to exposure. Vegetarians have to watch out, too, since MSG can be hidden in "vegetable proteins" that are often substituted for meats. And of course, diet sodas containing aspartame are OUT!

A great source of information on this topic is Russell Blaylock's book *Excitotoxins: The Taste That Kills* and his website www.russellblaylockmd.com.

NUTRITION TIP #7: AVOID UNHEALTHY FATS, EAT HEALTHY FATS

If you remember in our conversation about supplements for brain health, we learned the importance of the omega-3 essential fatty acids EPA and DHA. Yes, it can be helpful to supplement with these fatty acids because it's easier to get higher daily therapeutic doses that way, and because of their anti-inflammatory and brain-sup-porting role, higher doses are good. Having said that, there are also dietary choices that you can make that will bring healthy "good" fats instead of unhealthy "bad" fats.

Good fats are typically unsaturated fats. They include the omega-3s, and monounsaturated and polyunsaturated fats.

Monounsaturated fats include olive oil, canola oil, most nuts (such as almonds and hazelnuts), sesame oil, sunflower oil, olives and avocados. Polyunsaturated fats include walnuts, corn/soybean/safflower oil, sunflower and pumpkin seeds, flax seeds, fatty fish and tofu.

I do not condone all of those oils, because in some cases, such as corn, soy and canola oil, the oil will come from nuts and grains that are genetically modified, and that is not a good thing either. Genetically modified foods can mess with our DNA, and it is believed that they contribute to a lot of chronic disease in our society. I recommend at least one tablespoon of flax oil per day, and three servings of a wild caught fatty fish per week. I understand that there is some dilemma here with regards to fish and the potential heavy metal intake that comes with it, but I believe that three servings a week of a wild-caught, lower mercury level fish, such as salmon, is beneficial to one's health and outweighs the risk. I do not recommend farmed fish as they are typically fed grain, which changes the composition of their "healthy fats," and they do not contain the same nutrient profile. For example, pink coloring is often added to farmed salmon to make it look like salmon!

Trans fats and saturated fats are the bad fats. They are complete "brain blockers." They restrict healthy brain function and, in the long run, will be potentially life-threatening through their negative impact on cholesterol deposits, membrane permeability and oxidative damage. Saturated fats include meats, full fat dairy products, butter, palm oil, coconut oil and lard. Trans fats are generally created from man-made, processed foods: pizza, cookies, muffins, crackers, French fries, candy bars, pies and margarine. That list is endless, and unfortunately, these foods are so prevalent in the Western diet.

There are only two things that I would say are an exception to the rule that all saturated fats are evil. The first is grass-fed meat, which can have a healthier fatty acid profile. Back when bison roamed the prairie, their meat was very high in omega-3 fats. Today, because meat supply is big business, animals are fed grains, hormones and antibiotics, anything to fatten them up and produce more meat. In doing this, the fatty acid profile has taken a turn for the worse, and now the fat in most meat is saturated. Having said this, I do not have people remove red meat from their diet completely; I instead emphasize the importance of eating grass-fed meat. White meats such as chicken and turkey have lower saturated fat profiles but still need to be organic/free range so that they do not provide a source of hormones and antibiotics.

The second saturated fat is coconut oil. Coconut oil has received lots of attention in recent years for its health properties, and yet it is a saturated fat. How does that work? Well, coconut oil contains medium-chain triglycerides, which have many health-giving properties. They help to support a healthy metabolism, promote weight loss, support the immune system, support the thyroid gland and are healthy for the heart, amongst other things. Coconut oil contains lauric acid, which converts to monolaurin, which has antiviral and antimicrobial effects in the body. Caprylic acid is another constituent, and this has antifungal properties. Coconut oil is a very usable form of energy. The medium chain triglycerides in coconut oil are converted into ketones in the liver, providing an easily accessible energy source for organs and the brain. Because of this, the fatty acids in coconut oil are less likely to be stored as fat in adipose cells. It can be a better source of energy than sugar, with its corresponding spikes in blood glucose and insulin levels (which can, in excess, be harmful to the brain).

I advise having some coconut oil every day. I blend up a tablespoon of coconut oil or MCT oil (a derivative of coconut oil) in my smoothie sometimes, and that tastes really good. I have to admit that I have a latte each morning, and a tablespoon of coconut oil makes that creamy and yummy. Coconut oil is the best oil to cook with, too (even better than olive oil), because it is stable at high temperatures. I love olive oil raw, in salad dressings for example, but it will denature during cooking, changing its composition and making it potentially harmful. Coconut oil will retain its chemical makeup, so it is great for stir fries, steamed vegetables and sautéed meats and fish.

The fats that you eat can make a huge difference to your overall health and especially your brain health. Fish and flax are probably the two most direct sources of omega-3 fatty acids. Raw nuts and seeds are good sources of monounsaturated fats. Coconut oil is one of the best choices of all, given its use as an easy energy source for the body and its antimicrobial properties.

The brain is 60% fat. You are what you eat. If you eat horrible saturated and trans fats, that is what your brain will have to use as fuel and raw materials for cells and tissues. If you provide your body with healthy fatty acids through your diet, your brain will be able to utilize them, giving you healthier neurons, better blood supply, more flexible cell membranes and a less inflamed state. So stock up on flax oil, fish, olives, avocados, raw nuts and seeds, and lots of coconut oil, and enjoy a healthier brain!

NUTRITION TIP #8: EAT HIGH QUALITY, LEAN PROTEINS

This tip overlaps slightly with the previous one where we discussed some different types of meat, poultry and seafood as it relates to their fat content and composition.

Generally speaking, I am a supporter of high quality proteins in the diet, including meat, fish, turkey and chicken. I would recommend more of the fish and white meat than the red meat, but there is a place for all of them.

There are a few reasons to ensure you are getting adequate protein. Proteins are broken down to amino acids through the process of digestion. Amino acids are the building blocks of all our cells and tissues. When the body is damaged, it requires more amino acids to heal and rebuild. Proteins are needed in the brain to produce neurotransmitters, which as we know by now are formative for healthy brain structure and function, cognitive function and mood. Sometimes we will need to supplement with those particular amino acids to get a high enough boost for therapeutic effect, but making sure there are high quality proteins in the diet is a good starting point. A good example is when I steer a patient away from eating toast or cereal for breakfast and instead have them drink a high quality protein smoothie. Nine times out of ten, they will report that their cognitive function and alertness are improved throughout the entire day.

Animal proteins and seafood are also the highest dietary sources of vitamin B12. Mushrooms contain some (as do nuts) but not a significant amount. Dairy products do, too, but many Lyme patients (quite rightly) avoid dairy. Products such as tofu and soymilk are fortified with B12, but it is not naturally occurring in those foods. We know that B12 is one of the key nutrients for brain health, per our discussion on B12 supplementation, so it is important to make sure that adequate B12 levels are reached.

Liver has perhaps the highest B12 level of all (ewww!). Shellfish contain high levels of B12; clams, oysters, mussels and crab are the highest. Herring, mackerel, salmon, and tuna are also good sources. Red meat contains moderate amounts, while the amount in white meat, such as chicken and turkey, are relatively low.

For vegetarians, there may be even more reason to consider B12 supplementation, preferably via injection, since this is such an important brain-promoting nutrient.

Once again, I will stress the importance of grass-fed meats, organic poultry and wild-caught fish. Proteins are important for the body and the brain, but if they come with chemicals, hormones, antibiotics and unhealthy fatty acid profiles, they can do damage at the same time. People with Lyme Brain may be more susceptible to the deleterious effects of these additives, so keeping the protein sources pure and unadulterated will provide the best benefit in overcoming Lyme Brain.

NUTRITION TIP #9: DRINK WATER, WATER AND MORE WATER

We've talked a lot about what foods to put in your mouth to help your Lyme Brain, so let's touch on what drinks are best for you. Essentially, water is going to be your best ally in assisting brain function, because drinking water and optimal brain function are integrally linked. Lack of hydration to the brain is associated with memory issues, poor focus and concentration, depression, headaches, irritability and dizziness, and the list goes on. Water is needed to maintain healthy membranes for nerve transmission; it stops the brain from overheating; it helps flush toxins from the cells; and it improves blood circulation and, hence, oxygenation of tissues.

We lose approximately 80 ounces per day of water simply through sweating, breathing and metabolizing wastes. We also lose water overnight, even though sleeping may not seem like a very energetic activity. Therefore, we need to start our day with a large glass of pure, clean water, preferably with either the juice of a lemon or a few drops of lemon essential oil added. It will help to rehydrate the brain after our overnight "fast."

Researchers at the University of East London did an experiment on 34 men and women who fasted overnight and then were given either a cereal bar for breakfast or a cereal bar washed down with a bottle of water. Those who reported thirst, then were given the water, experienced a 14% improvement in their reaction times on a battery of mental tests that had been given once before the meal and again afterwards. They also found that children who drank water before a test fared up to a third better on their test scores.[11]

Thirst is certainly an indicator of physiological need for water as was shown in this study. However, dehydration can occur even before thirst is felt. That is why we must be proactive in our water intake. I have some patients who set a timer or alarm to drink a glass of water every two hours; otherwise, they won't do it. Water needs to be scheduled, just like medications and supplements need to be scheduled. Lyme Brain will be exacerbated without it.

NUTRITION TIP #10: AVOID DRINKING CAFFEINE AND ALCOHOL

As far as alcohol goes, I don't think I need to say much. For starters, the majority of Lyme sufferers simply cannot tolerate alcohol. One glass of wine and they will wake up the following day feeling like a college student in a frat house—hung over and terrible.

Beer is strongly discouraged because of its gluten content as well as its high yeast content.

It is no secret that alcohol blunts cognitive function, slows reflexes and mental responses, impacts memory and recall, and can fuel both depression and anxiety. It does everything to the brain that people with Lyme Brain want to avoid.

Further, there are several medications prescribed for Lyme and related co-infections that are absolutely contraindicated with alcohol. Rifampin and Tinidazole/Flagyl are two that come to mind. But realistically, alcohol is not a good idea with any antibiotic. Not only are there cross reactions and cumulative liver toxicity to consider, but in fighting the yeast fight that arises with long-term antibiotic use, adding alcohol to the mix is not a sensible choice.

There have been certain times when I have told a patient that they can enjoy a glass of wine here and there if they're out for dinner. Typically, as patients recover, they start looking for normalcy in their lives, and for some patients, having a sense of normalcy helps them stay on track in treatment. If it's a celebration or a special occasion and they have enough Lyme recovery under their belt already, then maybe. But that is more the exception to the rule. Most patients need to avoid alcohol entirely.

Alcohol is dehydrating, dulls the brain and the senses, feeds yeast overgrowth and contributes an unnecessary source of sugar. Alcohol mimics Lyme Brain and feeds it as well. It is best to avoid it.

In addition to alcohol, I frequently get questions about coffee and other caffeinated drinks. Now, the evidence on this one is mixed, and I am just giving my opinion based on the whole picture, not just on caffeine and brain function itself.

Caffeine is probably the most widely used psychoactive substance on the planet. It acts as a stimulant to the central nervous system. Certainly, there are many studies that validate increases in cognitive performance, short-term memory, recall, processing speeds and arousal. I am not denying that plenty of evidence exists to support that. So why wouldn't we use caffeine as a mental stimulant? It's cheap, it's legal and it doesn't require a prescription. What's not to love?

It is my opinion that there are some down sides to caffeine consumption that make it a slippery slope and not quite as ideal as all that.

For one, caffeine is a stimulant, so for many people that can lead to anxiety, irritability, jitters, sweating, trembling and insomnia. This is largely a dose-dependent response with everyone having different levels of sensitivity. Some people do fine with one cup, but if they were to have three cups, they would experience this kind of response. Many of my Lyme patients cannot tolerate any caffeine at all. Their nervous system is already on overdrive; they don't need any more hyperarousal.

Habituation is another issue. Basically, one cup might give a great brain-boosting effect for a while, but then it'll fade, and it will take two cups to have that same effect. The body adapts, and more and more of the substance is needed for the same benefit (this is really true of any addictive substance). Athletes also use caffeine to boost performance, but they have to use it selectively so that it works when they need it to work. I would suggest that the same is true for people with Lyme Brain. Caffeine is better saved for special occasions or moments of particular need so that it can be relied on to have the desired effect. In other words, if you have a meeting at work or a day where you need to focus on getting a lot of tasks done, drink caffeine then, but avoid it on days that you are at home with not much on your agenda, *even if you feel that you need it on those days.*

For those who are housebound, I would just avoid it altogether. Your nervous system has enough to deal with without having to process a stimulant. Caffeine is also dehydrating, so per our previous conversation about the benefits of water and adequate hydration, caffeine can set you back in that department.

What about green tea? Isn't that a good source of antioxidants? Well, yes, it is. And green tea also has lower caffeine levels than coffee. But to stay really kind to your nervous system, find a decaffeinated green tea or green tea extract and get the benefit without the caffeine.

Another major detriment of caffeine, and one of my major objections to it, is its impact on the adrenals. One cup of coffee a day might not be the end of the world, but people who use caffeine just to function and get through the day will ultimately put extra stress on their adrenal glands, which could lead them to even deeper exhaustion levels in the long term. The short-term gain may well not be worth the long-term damage. I am fully aware of the temptation to use caffeine to fuel the body when it is completely exhausted. However, a better, healthier way would be to work on rebuilding the adrenals and to work on the mitochondrial function of the cells so that the body can experience more internal, organic energy and not be as reliant on external crutches.

The next section is not directly related to nutrition, but while we're on the subject of coffee, let's talk about…

COFFEE ENEMAS

Yes, coffee enemas. For Lyme Brain!

I just gave you several good reasons why you should avoid caffeinated drinks, and then here I am talking about doing coffee enemas. Let me just clarify that most of the negative effects of drinking caffeine do not apply when using it for enemas; in fact, it often has the opposite effect. Therefore, the previous section applies to caffeinated drinks only, and the following information applies to enemas only.

More and more of my patients are using coffee enemas as a detox tool and find that it provides great relief. They are especially good during times of Herxing, as they do help to clear toxins from the body, but many use them on a regular basis, as frequently as every day.

Fans of coffee enemas report better sleep, more energy, better mood and certainly a clearer head. I have more than a few patients who use them as a pain-relief tool and find that they help stave off headaches and migraines. It might be a stretch to see how doing a coffee enema can help Lyme Brain. However, when you understand how it works, it does make sense.

Coffee enemas work in a couple of different ways. Coffee contains palmitic acids (kaweol and cafestol palmitate) that enhance glutathione-S-transferase in the liver, part of the enzyme system that functions in detoxification. The water in the enema enhances peristalsis, allowing for the movement of waste through the intestines and out through the anus.

Central to the process is that the fluid is absorbed through the intestinal wall and through the portal vein to the liver. It causes a stimulating effect on the liver and gall bladder, stimulating bile flow and allowing for a rapid dump and subsequent elimination of toxins. This is why people feel radically different immediately after a coffee enema. Very few things will provoke that much detox that rapidly without causing horrible detox side effects. Constituents in the coffee enhance bile flow and help it to move out of the bowel without being reabsorbed through the gut wall.

Further, coffee enemas enhance the production of glutathione itself. We have already discussed how important glutathione is for the brain and how to supplement it most effectively. Coffee enemas are another way to increase endogenous glutathione production.

Coffee enemas may also help clear parasites and Candida from the bowel. I have had some patients give graphic accounts of what landed in their toilet after an enema! If one has an overgrowth of such pathogens, coffee enemas can literally help sweep them out of the bowel.

While coffee enemas may seem a bit out there, they have a long history of use in both traditional and allopathic medical systems. They were even listed in the Merck Manual, a physician's handbook, until the mid-80s. Dr. Gerson is one of the key proponents of coffee enemas in his unique cancer protocol. He uses them alongside juicing, nutritional supplements and a special diet. In his protocol, however, people do several enemas per day, which I am not suggesting!

I personally do not recommend that people do more than one coffee enema per day. Some do every other day or twice weekly. Others save it for when they feel that they need more detox support, such as during Herxheimer reactions. I think daily coffee enemas are ideal for those who have the time and wherewithal to do them, and if that's not practical, one or two per week is better than nothing.

How are coffee enemas different from drinking coffee? They really do have different effects. Most people will experience drinking coffee as a sympathetic nervous system stimulant, making them jittery and anxious. Coffee enemas seem to act in the opposite way, enhancing the parasympathetic nervous system and acting as a relaxant (I've had a few patients for whom this was not the case, but it is in the majority of cases). Also, introducing the coffee into the intestines puts it directly in the portal circulatory system, meaning it goes directly to the liver rather than being circulated through the entire blood stream.

Coffee enemas may not be everyone's favorite activity! However, I have repeatedly seen the benefits when my patients got brave and gave them a try. The ability of coffee to cause the dilation of bile ducts, the increase in bile flow coupled with the enhancement of detox-related enzyme systems, the increase in endogenous glutathione production and the accelerated transit time out of the bowel all make for a pretty radical detoxification effect. This, in turn, promotes clearer thinking, improves mood and enhances sleep, all things that people with Lyme Brain crave.

REFERENCES

[1] Montagne, Axel, et al. "Blood-Brain Barrier Breakdown in the Aging Human Hippocampus." *Neuron* 85, no. 2 (January 2015): 296-302.

[2] Karakula-Juchnowicz, H, et al. "The role of IgG hypersensitivity in the pathogenesis and therapy of depressive disorders." *Nutr Neurosci.* 2014 30-September.

[3] Jackson, Jessica R, William W Eaton, Nicola G Cascella, Alessio Fasano, and Deanna L Kelly. "Neurologic and Psychiatric Manifestations of Celiac Disease and Gluten Sensitivity." *Psychiatr Q* 83, no. 1 (March 2012): 91-102.

[4] Hadjivassiliou, M, D S Sanders, R A Grunewald, N Woodroofe, S Boscolo, and D Aeschlimann. "Gluten sensitivity: from gut to brain." *Lancet Neurol* 9, no. 3 (March 2010): 318-30.

[5] Hadjivassiliou, M, et al. "Clinical, radiological, neurophysiological, and neuropathological characteristics of gluten ataxia." *Lancet* 352, no. 9140 (November 1998): 1582-5.

[6] Braniste, V, et al. "The gut microbiota influences blood-brain barrier permeability in mice." *Sci Transl Med* 6, no. 263 (November 2014): 263ra158.

[7] Agrawal, R, and F Gomez-Pinilla. "'Metabolic syndrome' in the brain: deficiency in omega-3 fatty acid exacerbates dysfunctions in insulin receptor signalling and cognition." *J Physiol* 590, no. Pt 10 (May 2012): 2485-99.

[8] Rabbitt, P, et al. "Losses in gross brain volume and cerebral blood flow account for age-related differences in speed but not in fluid intelligence." *Neuropsychology* 20, no. 5 (September 2006): 549-57.

[9] Crane, P K, et al. "Glucose levels and risk of dementia." *N Engl J Med* 369, no. 6 (August 2013): 540-8.

[10] Liu, Y, R Mittal, N V Solis, N V Prasadarao, and S G Filler. "Mechanisms of Candida albicans Trafficking to the Brain." *PLoS Pathog* 7, no. 10 (2011): e1002305.

[11] Edmonds, Caroline J, Rosanna Crombie, and Mark R Gardner. "Subjective thirst moderates changes in speed of responding associated with water consumption." *Front Hum Neurosci*, July 2013.

SECTION 5:

LIFESTYLE FACTORS

CHAPTER 20

SLEEP

—◦✕◦—

Sleep may be one of the most important factors in both helping Lyme Brain and recovering from Lyme disease, yet so many patients suffer from insomnia as part of their symptom picture. This sets up a real catch-22; sleep would help recovery from the disease, but the disease is preventing one from getting sleep. Sleep disturbances can range from trouble falling asleep, to non-restorative sleep, to waking at 2 a.m. and being unable to get back to sleep, to a complete reversal in circadian rhythms where one is awake most of the night and asleep during the day. Sleep apnea is also a fairly common problem amongst Lyme patients. Most of my patients would love to get more refreshing and regulated sleep, so just telling them to sleep more is futile and frustrating for them. Most would if they could.

There is a lot of research on the effects of lack of sleep on cognition. It has long been recognized that sleep deprivation leads to slower response speeds, less alertness, less vigilance and poor performance on tasks and tests. Emotional state is impacted by sleep deficit, as is motor performance. There is also evidence that sleep deprivation impacts higher-level cognitive functions such as executive functions, memory and perception. Sleep deprivation is associated with a higher risk of accidents.[1, 2]

It is recognized that Lyme patients have a particularly bad issue with sleep. One sleep study[3] examined a cohort of Lyme patients against age-matched normal controls. It compared polysomnographic measures of sleep between two groups over a two-night period. Multiple sleep latency testing (a series of scheduled naps or sleep periods in a prescribed period of time) was also performed on both groups. All patients experienced sleep-related complaints including trouble falling asleep, nighttime waking, restless leg syndrome and daytime sleepiness. However, in the Lyme patients, there was a longer sleep latency (the time taken from lying down to falling asleep), decreased sleep efficiency and higher arousal index (greater interruptions in sleep).

There are two types of sleep: REM sleep and non-REM sleep. REM sleep accounts for approximately 20% of total sleep; this is when dreaming occurs. Non-REM sleep is categorized as stage 1 and 2, or light sleep, and stage 3 and 4 is known as slow wave or deep sleep. Eighty percent of our sleep is non-REM sleep, and about 10-20% is slow wave sleep. The transition between REM and non-REM sleep is also largely driven by neurons in the brainstem and neurotransmitter release. It is purported that Lyme patients have a reduction in slow wave sleep, which is the type that is vital for the body to repair and regenerate.

The sleep study cited previously found that Lyme patients had more interruptions in stage 2 and stage 4 non-REM sleep, indicating more fragmented sleep. This study demonstrates the greater severity of common sleep issues in Lyme patients, which can contribute greatly to Lyme Brain.

Why are Lyme patients hit so hard in the area of sleep? Sleep is regulated by several areas and aspects of the brain. Parts of the brainstem and hypothalamus send arousal signals to the cerebral cortex to promote wakefulness, and much of this occurs via neurotransmitter transmission. Another area of the hypothalamus is responsible for shutting down the body's arousal signals and promoting the transition to sleep. The pineal gland secretes melatonin, which helps to regulate our sleep and wake cycles. The body naturally produces more melatonin around nighttime (or at least it is supposed to!) and lower amounts during the day. Darkness will prompt the body to produce more melatonin, while light will lead to less of it.

We have already seen the extent to which chronic infections can cause an immune cascade, which includes immune chemicals such as cytokines and chemokines. Such inflammatory chemicals can also impact the parts of the brain that regulate sleep patterns. Thus, at the same time as trying to find ways to help sleep directly, we still must work on reducing the infectious load and reducing inflammation in the body to get lasting results.

In summary, Lyme can impact both the homeostatic mechanisms of the body, such as the hypothalamic regulation of sleep, and it can impact the hypothalamus-pituitary-adrenal axis, which completely messes with hormonal regulation of sleep.

I also see many patients who wake around 2 a.m. nightly often take a few hours to fall back to sleep or not fall back to sleep at all. While this may be a Lyme issue, I also believe that Candida overgrowth can contribute as well. If you recall from our earlier conversation, Candida produces acetaldehydes that act like alcohol in the brain and can be great sleep interrupters. I have also seen the co-infection Babesia cause a lot of sleep problems. A broad-spectrum antimicrobial protocol is necessary to address the range of infections that may be playing a role.

Elevated cortisol at night can be another contributor to poor sleep quality. This is related to the disturbance of the hypothalamic-pituitary-adrenal axis, as cortisol is the stress hormone produced by your adrenal glands. It is supposed to be highest in the morning to energize you and then drop progressively throughout the course of the day to its lowest level at night. This allows your immune system to kick in at night and do its housekeeping work, which is vital to recovery from Lyme. If cortisol is elevated at night, it can cause hyperarousal and insomnia. Salivary adrenal testing is the best way to assess this, because it measures cortisol in the morning, at noon, in the afternoon and at night. It is interesting to see the imbalances that can occur during the day. Sometimes morning cortisol levels are just fine, but then they dip low in the afternoon causing an energy lull and/or spike at night causing the insomnia issue. A standard blood test showing morning cortisol only could miss this whole dynamic and, subsequently, a vital opportunity to help modulate sleep patterns.

There are a few simple things that one can do at home to support healthy sleep patterns. Sometimes it is necessary to take prescription sleep medication for a period of time just to give the body some rest and recovery time. While that is not ideal, there are times when chronic sleep deprivation can be so damaging to the body that the risk is worth it.

Here are some ideas that can help with sleep:

❖ Install blackout shades or curtains to ensure total darkness.

❖ Go to bed at the same time every night and get up at the same time every day. The more sleep one gets before midnight, the better, so 10 p.m.–5 a.m. is better than 12 p.m.–7 a.m. in terms of recovery. Try to train the body into a routine.

❖ Avoid any stimulants such as caffeine. Some people will experience sleep disturbance even from caffeine taken in the morning.

❖ Avoid alcohol and sugar.

❖ Make sure to eat your last meal at least three hours before bedtime so you're not going to bed on a full stomach.

❖ Remove any devices from your bedroom that are Wi-Fi or Bluetooth and have as few devices plugged into electrical outlets as possible. I have had numerous patients report improvements in sleep once they left their cell phones, iPads, etc. in the kitchen overnight, and even when they switched out their clock radio for a regular clock.

Supplements that can help sleep:

Melatonin – melatonin is a commonly used supplement to assist with sleep. As mentioned, melatonin is a substance produced by the pineal gland that naturally regulates night and day/dark and light cycles. In my opinion, melatonin is generally quite safe and can be effective for some, especially in the realm of falling asleep. Unfortunately, it has a short duration of action in the body, and so it is not as helpful for staying asleep. Thankfully, there is a prolonged-release form that is better for helping to stay asleep. Many people will take both so that one can help them fall asleep and the other will release gradually to help them stay asleep.

5-HTP – we talked about 5-HTP in the section on amino acids as an aid for depression and anxiety. 5-HTP converts to serotonin, which then converts to melatonin. Some people find 5-HTP works better for them than melatonin, but it does need to be taken in higher doses (approximately 200mg) to get the sleep benefit. Conversely, if people take it during the day for depression but take too high of a dose for them, they will experience sleepiness. It can take some time to figure out the best schedule and dose for you.

Herbs – valerian, California poppy and passionflower are some of the herbs that can help with sleep. Valerian is one of the most common and often works well, except that there are some people who have the total opposite reaction to it and become "wired."

Phosphatidylserine and adaptogenic herbs for the adrenals – as previously discussed, phosphatidylserine can be very helpful for reducing abnormally high levels of cortisol. A 50–100mg dose taken just before dinner can help balance levels by bedtime. I usually use phosphatidylserine along with other balancing herbs for the adrenals. Adaptogenic herbs, by definition, will lower elevated levels and boost low levels; they are balancing to the system. Herbs such as ashwaghanda and rhodiola fall into that category.

I have developed a sleep formula called Dr. Nicola's Sleep Support capsules with which I've had tremendous results. I always joke that it contains every natural sleep aid known to man, and that's not far from the truth. It's a very comprehensive formula that I have found works much better than any single supplement alone. Its ingredients are 5-HTP, melatonin, theanine, valerian, GABA, inositol, passionflower, hops, chamomile, California poppy, Jamaican dogwood, skullcap, hops, jujube seed and wild lettuce leaf (available from www.restormedicine.com).

In terms of medications, one of my favorites is trazadone. Trazadone is an old-school antidepressant medication, but because there are so many newer generations of antidepressants now, it is mostly prescribed for sleep. I like it because it is not habit forming as many others are. It also helps promote the deeper stages of sleep—Stage 3 and 4 non-REM sleep. Zyrem is another medication that does this, but it is a stronger medication with more side effects. The most common side effects I see with trazadone are a dry mouth in the morning and vivid dreams. Some find Lyrica very helpful for sleep quality as well as nerve pain. Yet others find that antihistamines will have a sufficiently sedating effect; Doxafin is an example of this. People, however, should avoid wherever possible taking benzodiazepines, such as clonazepam, to assist their sleep. These medications are highly habit forming and can be brutal to wean off.

I understand that many Lyme patients are indeed taking these kinds of medications for insomnia and anxiety, and in some cases, they have tried other things without any benefit at all, but I always encourage patients to start with the least invasive and work their way up from there.

Another modality that I find very helpful for insomnia is neurofeedback, which we will discuss more in the next section.

Clearly, insomnia is a far-reaching problem for many Lyme patients. It is so important to correct imbalances in sleep patterns given the direct correlation between sleep disturbance and cognitive deficits. It is also important in the grand scheme of recovery, as sleep is vital to the body's repair and regeneration process.

REFERENCES

[1] Centers for Disease Control and Prevention. *Autism Spectrum Disorder (ASD) Data & Statistics.* 2000-2010. http://www.cdc.gov/ncbddd/autism/data.html.

[2] Kessler, R C, W T Chiu, O Demler, K R Merikangas, and E E Walters. "Prevalence, severity, and comorbidity of 12-month DSM-IV disorders in the National Comorbidity Survey Replication." *Arch Gen Psychiatry* 62, no. 6 (July 2005): 617-27.

[3] Greenberg, Rosalie. "Tick-Borne Diseases and the Brain: Implications for Pediatric Psychiatry." *ILADS Conference 2014.* Washington, DC, October 10th, 2014.

CHAPTER 21

EXERCISE

⸺⸺◁✕▷⸺⸺

Generally speaking, exercise can provide huge benefits for cognitive function. It also functions as an anti-anxiety and antidepressive modality. Research clearly shows the benefit to cognitive function of regular exercise, especially frontal lobe-mediated activities such as planning, scheduling, inhibition and working memory.[1]

There are a few different mechanisms for this. It seems that brain neurons increase in number with just days or weeks of regular aerobic exercise. MRI studies of a group of adults over 55 years of age showed that there were natural age-related losses of brain tissue density and volume, but that those losses could be offset by regular physical activity and correlated with cardiovascular fitness.[2] In another study of 1,740 adults older than 65, the incidence of dementia was 35% lower in individuals who walked three times a week or more.[3]

Exercise also helps to boost blood flow and oxygenation to the brain. It upregulates mitochondrial functioning and neuronal metabolic state. This enhancement in metabolism in the brain is mediated in part by a substance called brain-derived neurotrophic factor (BDNF). BDNF, which works as a metabotrophin (a promoter of metabolism), is associated with the upregulation of a range of other substances that influence energy and synaptic plasticity. The result of one study showed that when exercise-induced BDNF was suppressed, there was a correlated decline in spatial learning and memory that had been enhanced during exercise protocols otherwise.[4]

Neurotropic factors that are stimulated by exercise can also promote neurogenesis (creation of new neurons), giving it an even greater importance.

Another way that exercise helps cognitive function is by reducing reactive oxygen species in the brain. Reactive oxygen species are the products of aerobic metabolism (which happens in our cells as a product of normal

159

metabolism), and they are what we think of as "oxidants." The brain is particularly vulnerable to reactive oxygen species. We have talked a lot so far about various supplements that can act as antioxidants in the brain. As it turns out, exercise can help reduce oxidative stress on the brain and, therefore, act as an antioxidant itself. By modulating this oxidative state and relieving oxidative stress, which results in better functioning and improvements in factors such as active learning and memory.[5]

It appears that the type of exercise makes a difference in how it impacts cognition. One study[6] divided a cohort of older women with mild cognitive impairment into three groups: some did aerobic exercise, some did weight training, and the third group stretched and toned only. At the end of six months, they performed a battery of tests to assess not only memory, but different types of memory such as verbal, spatial and associative. The women in the toning group performed worse on their cognitive tests than their baseline, indicating that their cognitive decline had not been positively impacted by their activity. Both the weight training group and the aerobic activity group performed better on spatial memory. Interestingly, though, there were still differences between those two groups. The aerobic exercise group also improved in verbal memory whereas the weight-training group did not. This indicates that different types of exercise impact different parts of the brain and different brain functions.

Another study on exercise and memory demonstrated similar findings.[7] In this study, rats either ran on a treadmill or lifted weights (not so easy to set up, I'm sure, but apparently they tied weights to their tails and made them climb little ladders to stimulate resistance training, poor little rats). The runner rats demonstrated an increase in BDNF (which as mentioned earlier, supports healthy neurons and the production of new neurons) while the weight-training group did not. However, they showed higher levels of insulin-like growth factor (IGF), which supports healthy cell division and growth, and protects new neurons. The net result was that both groups had improvements in learning and spatial memory. However, the mechanism was slightly different based on the type of exercise.

It is not just older adults who show benefits of exercise for their brain. Children have higher test scores and a greater ability to concentrate when they get regular exercise.

Another major benefit of exercise is a reduction in depression and anxiety. Exercise has a positive impact on neurotransmitter production, including the serotonergic, dopaminergic and noradrenergic systems. It has also been found that the insulin-like growth factor and BDNF have positive impacts on depressive states as well as cognition.[8]

So how does this all relate to Lyme patients? I can already hear some of you saying, "Well that's all lovely, but I can't even get out of bed." Yes, I understand. There are many people who are bedbound and/or homebound, riddled with pain and completely exhausted. Any kind of regular exercise may not be a realistic idea… yet! It's a bit like the sleep issue. I'm sure if you could sleep more you would, but it seems elusive. A 30-minute walk outside might seem a world away from where you are right now. However, I would offer two things by way of encouragement.

First, if you are severely debilitated and unable to do any aerobic exercise, still try to do some mild gentle weight training as a starting point. It helps to rehabilitate the muscles and, most importantly, still triggers the BDNF and IGF, which help support healthy neurons and can positively impact cognition and mood. That might mean lifting a tin can a few times in the beginning. Second, you can look forward to incorporating more aerobic activity once you get a little further along in your recovery. Just keep in mind for the time being how important it is and how much it will be able to help you in the future.

Lyme patients function at various levels. Some of my patients are still working full-time jobs, raising children, single parenting and/or are the breadwinners of the family. Some have to force themselves out of necessity while some are well enough to maintain a high level of normalcy in their lives. Some are keeping up regular exercise regimens while others are unable to do anything consistently.

For those who can, I am a believer in doing some aerobic exercise as well as some light weight training. I don't mean that you should run five miles every day or do triathlons. However, I do suggest that you do at least 20 minutes at least three times weekly in a manner that raises the heart rate. I view walking and swimming as two optimal types of exercise. A steady stationary bike is good, too. Patients with POTS-type presentations may benefit most from a seated type of exercise such as a recumbent bike or rowing machine. I find that many of my patients benefit greatly from the stress-relieving aspects, and it helps them stay connected to what they love to do in their lives. As a runner myself, I know I would feel that way. If I were facing health challenges, I would still try to keep up some kind of exercise regimen, even if I had to tone it down from what it used to be. It would be better for my mental health to do that than to have to quit altogether. I have many patients who feel the same way.

My rule of thumb is this: If you do a certain exercise and feel tired afterwards but wake up the next day feeling back to baseline, then that is likely to be okay for your body. If you feel wiped out afterwards and wake the next day still exhausted, then that is a sign that whatever you are doing is too much. We must remember that too much exercise will strain the adrenal glands, which are already under stress due to chronic illness. Sometimes testing cortisol levels helps to determine an appropriate exercise regimen. If cortisol levels are very low, I would be more cautious about recommending exercise regimens. If cortisol levels are normal, then that can be an indicator that the body can handle exercise better. High cortisol is a sign that the body is in overdrive and is in a compensatory mode for chronic stressors. In these cases, too much exercise can be even more stimulating, and more gentle forms of exercise may be indicated.

Whatever your level of functioning and capability, doing some exercise is proven to be beneficial for the neurological system by increasing oxygenation and blood supply to the brain, helping the metabolism and mitochondrial function of cells and perhaps, most importantly, boosting both insulin-like growth factor and brain-derived neurotropic factor. The bottom line is this: even mild/gentle exercise as part of your recovery can help regenerate neurons and boost cognitive function.

REFERENCES

[1] Ratey, J J, and J F Loehr. "The positive impact of physical activity on cognition during adulthood: a review of underlying mechanisms, evidence and recommendations." Rev Neurosci 22, no. 2 (2011): 171-85.

[2] Colcombe, S J, et al. "Aerobic fitness reduces brain tissue loss in aging humans." J Gerontol A Biol Sci Med Sci 58, no. 2 (February 2003): 176-80.

[3] Larson, E B, et al. "Exercise is associated with reduced risk for incident dementia among persons 65 years of age and older." Ann Intern Med 144, no. 2 (January 2006): 73-81.

[4] Gomez-Pinilla, F, S Vaynman, and Z Ying. "Brain-derived neurotrophic factor functions as a metabotrophin to mediate the effects of exercise on cognition." Eur J Neurosci 28, no. 11 (December 2008): 2278-87.

[5] Radak, Z, S Kumagai, A W Taylor, H Naito, and S Goto. "Effects of exercise on brain function: role of free radicals." Appl Physiol Nutr Metab 32, no. 5 (October 2007): 942-6.

[6] Nagamatsu, L S, et al. "Physical activity improves verbal and spatial memory in older adults with probable mild cognitive impairment: a 6-month randomized controlled trial." J Aging Res 2013 (2013): 861893.

[7] Cassilhas, R C, et al. "Spatial memory is improved by aerobic and resistance exercise through divergent molecular mechanisms." Neurosience 202 (January 2012): 309-17.

[8] Paslakis, G, W F Blum, and M Deuschle. "Intranasal insulin-like growth factor I (IGF-I) as a plausible future treatment of depression." Med Hypotheses 79, no. 2 (August 2012): 222-5.

CHAPTER 22

EXERCISING THE BRAIN

———⊸⊲⊳⊶———

We have talked so far about the benefits of exercise and its effects on Lyme Brain. Exercising the brain itself can also be helpful, but how does one do that? By engaging in regular tasks that require memory, focus, decision-making, and learning and reasoning processes. This can be anything from playing memorization or matching games to crossword puzzles, Sudoku puzzles and commercial programs such as Lumosity.

Companies such as Lumosity, which offer computer-based cognitive training programs, are popping up everywhere. Brain training is becoming quite a large market. In fact, Lumosity claims to have 70 million people using their web-based product.

Their website cites multiple studies demonstrating cognitive improvements amongst a broad range of individuals, including adult and pediatric cancer survivors, girls with Turner syndrome (a genetic disorder which disrupts cognitive function and produces deficits in mathematical ability), neurotypical children, older adults, adults with mild cognitive impairment and healthy middle-aged adults.

The study done on breast cancer survivors was particularly interesting given that the study was also reflecting pathology that impacts brain function rather than simply age-related cognitive decline. Chemotherapy is known to impact cognition, which potentially lasts 10 to 20 years post-treatment. A standard neuropsychological test was given before and after the 12-week training period, during which half the women did Lumosity exercises and the other half did not. Exercises were based around working memory, processing speed, mental flexibility and verbal fluency. At the end of the 12-week period, the women who trained showed improved scores on the neuropsychological testing while the control group did not.[1]

However, there is also research that indicates the computerized training tools may not be as effective as some claim. In a 2014 review, researchers looked at 51 trials encompassing over 5000 subjects.[2] In analyzing all the data, they found that computerized cognitive training had a small but still statistically significant impact. So there was enough of a benefit to make it more than pure chance, but it was not a tremendous benefit. They also found that computerized training programs were likely to improve non-verbal memory (remembering visual images) and working memory (short-term memory and recent events) but did not seem to impact executive functions such as planning and judgment, or concentration and focus. Home-based programs were found to be less effective than programs run within facilities.

Some claim that the more effective brain-training exercises are actually those that involve daily life tasks, such as memorizing a shopping list, drawing places or items from memory, trying to recall a recipe with specific quantities of specific ingredients, and doing math sums in your head instead of using a calculator.

Other home-grown brain training activities may include creating word games (such as seeing how letters can be rearranged to form new words), learning a new language, taking up a new hobby to challenge different parts of the brain, performing activities that require fine motor skills such as crafting or sewing, and learning a new word from the dictionary every day. Other ideas include picking a city name that starts with each letter of the alphabet, writing with your non-dominant hand, and recalling items from yesterday's activities.

Remembering things by association can be very helpful, too. For instance, using acronyms to help remember items on lists (who didn't learn the colors of the rainbow by ROY G BIV?!). I know that I survived the early years of medical school by making up goofy stories around the words I was trying to memorize. It may sound silly, but it works! It is also helpful to arrange words on a page with different structures and different colors in order to remember them. That way, you can visualize where they are on the page or how they are written as opposed to just a generic list or a paragraph where nothing stands out. These small exercises need not take long and can be fun. It all helps.

Irrespective of the discrepancies in the research on the success of different modes of brain training and based on the premise of "use it or lose it," it makes sense to keep the brain active as much as possible. I know people who use programs such as Lumosity and love doing the exercises every day; its structure works for them. Others love the crossword puzzles or word games in the newspaper. Yet others just create little challenges for themselves throughout the day based on activities of daily living. Whatever works for you, I have heard from many patients that keeping their brain active helps them to overcome Lyme Brain. It also gives them a sense of empowerment knowing that they are working to keep their brain as healthy as possible.

REFERENCES

[1] Kesler, Shelli, et al. "Cognitive Training for Improving Executive Function in Chemotherapy-Treated Breast Cancer Survivors." *Clinical Breast Cancer* 13, no. 4 (August 2013): 299-306.

[2] Lampit, Amit, Harry Hallock, and Michael Valenzuela. "Computerized Cognitive Training in Cognitively Healthy Older Adults: A Systematic Review and Meta-Analysis of Effect Modifiers." *PLoS Medicine*, November 2014.

CHAPTER 23

THOUGHT LIFE

Some of you might get slightly irritated when I tell you to think positive thoughts and continue to give yourself positive messages of hope and recovery. But please hear me out. There is a reason why this is so crucial to your recovery.

That reason is neuroplasticity. Neuroplasticity is the brain's ability to adapt and change in response to its environment. That may occur in a number of ways for a number of reasons ranging from damage due to a stroke, to the thought patterns and beliefs we adopt.

It was once thought that the brain was a static entity. Neurons were set in number and once they died, that was it; no new ones could grow. It was also thought that the brain had very specific areas associated with very specific functions, and that if that area of the brain was damaged, then the function associated with it was also lost forever.

It is now emerging that these limited views of the brain are incorrect. New neurons *can* be created, and damaged neurons *can* be regenerated. Amazingly, when parts of the brain are damaged, other parts—parts that are not supposed to know how to do the tasks associated with that area—can take over and step in.

In *The Brain That Changes Itself*, Norman Doidge presents solid research as well as cases that demonstrate this. I highly recommend it if you are interested in this area of neuroplasticity. It is fascinating and amazing to hear how adaptable the brain is in the face of adversity. In the Lyme world, this principle still applies, but in a slightly different way. Because research shows that Lyme Brain is more about diffuse inflammatory, circulatory, metabolic and infectious processes rather than focal points of damage, we do not see as many cases where one small area of the brain is damaged and other parts take on the responsibility for those specific roles. This might be more relevant to stroke victims, for example, or head trauma victims, where damage is more localized.

However, neuroplasticity can still be of huge benefit to Lyme patients. It is important in the thoughts that we choose and the neural networks that we build up around these thoughts.

I used to think that the whole "positive thinking" movement and positive psychology was a bit of hooey. Just think positively and you will create positive outcomes in your life. It all sounded good, but without understanding the science of neuroplasticity, it sounded a bit hokey and unrealistic. Since learning about neuroplasticity and really "getting" how profound this is, I have implemented it in my own life (and have seen others do the same) with incredible results. Consider this: a thought is really an electrochemical reaction. It is a series of nerve cells transmitting impulses, with neurotransmitters in the synapses helping the transmission of the nerve along to the next neuron. Thoughts are "the result or product of either spontaneous or willed acts of thinking."[1] One thing we know about neurons is that repetition strengthens the neural connections that support whatever thought or activity is being repeated. To cite a really simple example, if you try to learn the lyrics to a song, you probably won't be able to remember them easily at first. Maybe you'll go line by line and repeat them to yourself a few words at a time until that line is locked in. Then you'll go on to the next line and try to remember those. By the time you have memorized the lyrics to the entire song, you'll have grown and strengthened the neural networks involved in that process. Next thing you know, you'll be driving down the road when that song comes on the radio. You'll consciously sing along while unconsciously remembering the words. Another example is learning to play a song on a musical instrument. It's very conscious and very deliberate in the beginning but once learned can become automatic.

An analogy I like to use is that of a small neuron dirt track that can grow into a neuronal superhighway. When you first try to remember the line, that neural pathway is like a small dirt track. It may barely fit one person walking it and there may be rocks, which make it hard to navigate. Not even a car can get down that dirt track. As time goes on and you practice more and more, that dirt track widens. Now a car can drive on it, and the rocks and bumps smooth out. More neurons are recruited to support the activity and process, and neural connections are strengthened. Even further along the process and the dirt track gets paved. Now one car can drive it comfortably. With more time, practice and repetition occurs, and now it's a two-lane road with traffic moving in both directions. Even further along, it continues to grow, and eventually it becomes a superhighway with eight lanes and traffic speeding along unimpeded. The only difference between the little dirt track neural pathway and the superhighway neural pathway is choice, practice and repetition. It has to be deliberate; it is not going to happen on its own. The neuronal superhighway now looks like a vast number of neurons all working together to support whatever activity is being practiced. Repetition makes it stronger, until that process is locked in.

So it is with thought patterns. A positive thought might start out like that little dirt track. It might even be hard to create that dirt track—you've been sick for so long, your marriage has fallen apart, you can't raise your children and be involved in their lives as you would like, you feel isolated, you've lost your friends, you have had to sell your home and move into a smaller place to pay all your medical bills; and yet, you still have huge credit card debt. Recovery seems hopeless. After all, you've been at it for years and you're still not better. I would encourage you to just do it. Choose a positive thought or idea, something hopeful about your healing or your life. Repeat it multiple times a day, preferably out loud. Realize that at first, it's going to be a little dirt track neuronal pathway. You have to *choose* to build it up into a proper paved road, then a two-lane highway and finally a superhighway. Picture that road building and growing. Be deliberate about it. It won't happen on its own by some automatic miracle; you need to work at it. It won't be easy at first, but as the neuronal pathways are strengthened, it will become easier. And finally, it will be automatic. You have programmed your neurological system to believe that thought until that thought becomes truth for you.

The bad news is that just as we can create neuronal pathways around positive healthy thoughts, we can just as easily create them around negative, pessimistic thoughts and emotions. The process is exactly the same. Caroline Leaf, Ph.D. is a researcher who has looked deeply into the role of toxic thinking on our health. She gives the following examples that might indicate that you are hosting toxic thoughts that can be detrimental to your health:

How many "could have," "would have," "should have" statements have you made today?

* ❖ How many "if onlys" were part of your inner vocabulary today?

* ❖ How many times have you replayed in your head a conversation or situation that pained you, or one that hasn't even occurred yet?

* ❖ How many scenarios have you created of the unpredictable future?

* ❖ How much time is speculation taking out of your day?

* ❖ How passive is your mind?

* ❖ How honest are you with yourself?

❖ Are you at cross purposes with yourself —going through the motions, but not really committed to the goal, saying one thing but meaning another?

❖ How distorted is your thinking? Are you forming a personal identity around for example, a disease? Do you speak about *my* arthritis, *my* multiple sclerosis, *my* heart problem?

❖ Do you ever make comments like "Nothing ever goes right for me", "Everything I touch fails" or "I always mess up"?

Dr. Leaf states that if the previous examples are a regular part of your daily thought life, your mind may need "detoxing." According to her, this is done by "learning to engage interactively with every single thought that you have and to analyze it before you decide either to accept or reject it."[2]

I love Dr. Leaf's work, and I would highly recommend her book *Switch on Your Brain: The Key to Peak Happiness, Thinking and Health*, which will expand on these ideas and give you real direction for change. She also wrote *Who Switched off Your Brain: Solving the Mystery of He Said/She Said*, which focuses on the difference between the male and female brains (what? there's a difference?!). For those who need help detoxing their negative thoughts, she also offers a program called the 21-day Brain Detox. She writes from a Christian perspective; her work is deeply rooted in science while being engaging and easy to read.

I find this whole body of work fascinating, and it can make a significant impact on your brain and your health. You have over 30,000 thoughts per day, and you create neural pathways all the time. You might as well make them positive ones.

CAN NEUROPLASTICITY OVERCOME GENETIC MAKEUP?

Neuroplasticity actually releases us from our genetic destiny.

Harvard Medical School's Dr. Alvaro Pascual-Leone recently stated that:

> "Neuroplasticity is an intrinsic property of the human brain and represents evolution's invention to enable the nervous system to escape the restrictions of its own genome and thus adapt to environmental pressures, physiological changes, and experiences."[3]

This statement implies that neuroplasticity allows us to overcome our genetics and adapt to environmental influences and experiences. The great part is that we get to choose many of those experiences.

Dr. Bruce Lipton discusses this at length in his lectures entitled "The Biology of Belief." While researching muscle cells, he found that muscle cells that come from the same muscle and therefore have the same DNA acted differently depending on the environment in which they were placed. How is this possible if DNA, aka genetics, dictates what controls the cell? He goes on to explain that, in truth, it is the environment that controls the cells. The environment interacts with the cell's receptors on its outer membrane. This triggers signaling proteins that cross the membrane into the cell, triggering yet other proteins within the cell. Those proteins will then go to the DNA and, depending on the need based on the environment, will create the proteins needed from the DNA template. The DNA is *responding* to the environmental milieu rather than *controlling* it.

This is a major paradigm shift from "we're a victim of our genetics" to "our genetics can be influenced by our environment" and it's really the outside influences, or *perceptions*, of the cell that regulate how its DNA is transcribed. This is very positive, as some people get stuck thinking that they're going to end up with a certain disease or health limitation because it runs in their family. Based on the work of Bruce Lipton and others, we are far more empowered than we might think to control and optimize our health by regulating our environment.

Let's look at that from a standpoint of thought and emotional life. The cell responds to environmental influences, and those influences include thoughts and emotions. When the cell is bombarded with negative thoughts and emotions, it can influence the health of the organism, including impacting its immune function, potentially leading to disease and dysfunction in the body.

Bruce Lipton, Ph.D. explains this phenomenon in detail (much better than I have!), and I would highly recommend his work. I like to listen to his lectures on YouTube (search *biology of belief*). If you're a reader, his book *The Biology of Belief: Unleashing the Power of Consciousness, Matter and Miracles* is a great starting point. He has also published a great audio CD titled *The Wisdom of Your Cells: How Your Beliefs Control Your Biology.*

This demonstrates that individual cells can be influenced by their environment and that we can influence the environment through good nutrition, minimizing toxicity, and regulating the thoughts and emotions to which the cell is exposed.

Thus we can see two significant things here. First, by choosing positive thoughts, we can create stronger neuronal pathways to support those thoughts until they become automatic, unconscious and considered truth by our system. And second, those positive thoughts then become part of the cellular environmental influence, which can influence how our genes are expressed through DNA and RNA transcription. This can then positively influence immune function and any other physiological process in the body.

REFERENCES

[1]"Thought." *Wikipedia*. December 18, 2015. https://en.wikipedia.org/wiki/Thought (accessed August 4th, 2015).

[2] Leaf, Caroline. "Controlling Your Toxic Thoughts." *Dr. Leaf.* 2016. http://drleaf.com/about/toxic-thoughts/.

[3] Pascual-Leone, A, A Amedi, F Fregni, and L B Merabet. "The plastic human brain cortex." *Annu Rev Neurosci* 28 (2005): 377-401.

CHAPTER 24

ADDRESSING PSYCHOEMOTIONAL
ISSUES AND TRAUMA

We have talked about the power of your thoughts and how to remove toxic thoughts from your brain, thus rewiring the brain in healthier patterns. However, there are certain thoughts and experiences that may be deeply entrenched in the subconscious, and it may be worthwhile to get counseling or some other kind of therapy to assist with those aspects. This can absolutely help with some of the anxiety and depression pieces but can also help with the cognitive and behavioral, too. Different types of therapy have different focuses and different strengths. Remember, too, that some of the depression and anxiety is infection related, meaning that the infections and ensuing inflammation are throwing off the neurological system and creating those symptoms. But some of the psychological and psychiatric symptoms may be underpinned by other dynamics that can be aided by therapy.

Many people have suffered great losses—marriages, careers, friendships and financial freedom, to name just a few—through their experience with Lyme. These losses can give rise to many emotions such as resentment, sadness, anger, regret, guilt, fear, shame, envy and hopelessness. So in this case, the underlying factor is one's reaction or response to the disease itself and all the destruction it has brought. I would say this is a pretty natural response to a terrible situation; however, living with those emotions will not serve any positive purpose, so overcoming them is valuable. Therapy can help you come to terms with some of these emotions so they are not hindering recovery. It is certainly true that a good therapist will offer emotional support in ways that might be hard for Lyme patients to find in their families, friends or communities. The value of that cannot be overstated.

Other people have other underlying issues that might be long-standing and possibly unrelated to their Lyme situation. The Lyme might make dealing with them harder, or they might just be coexisting. They may even be masked by the Lyme disease, which is so all-encompassing that there is no time and energy left to deal with much of anything else.

There are many types of therapy available, and different styles may work for different people. Here are just a few that I have been exposed to. However, this is just a tiny smattering of a very broad field.

COUNSELING/TALK THERAPY

Counseling is either a one-on-one or a group therapy process that centers on an individual talking through their thoughts, feelings and life circumstances in a way that provides introspection, self-awareness and transformation. Many times, by bringing something to light rather than suppressing it and ignoring it, it is easier to work through. Therapists can provide caring listening, emotional support and their own insights and feedback about the issues that are on the table.

In my experience, many people with Lyme disease benefit greatly from this kind of intervention, as not only can they work through underlying emotional roadblocks, but they feel a huge sense of relief to be listened to and well-supported, and not judged.

In my opinion, one of the limitations of this kind of therapy is that it can take quite a long time to reveal, discuss, and process emotions to the point that true change can occur. I have seen other kinds of therapy, such as energy psychology, affect change faster. However, I have great respect for the therapeutic process and relationship, and I have seen many Lyme patients benefit greatly from it.

COGNITIVE-BEHAVIORAL THERAPY

Cognitive-behavioral therapy can be very helpful for people with Lyme Brain, because it teaches skills and adaptive behaviors that can help overcome some of the deficits caused by the disease.

A cognitive-behavioral therapist will assess a patient to learn where maladaptive thought patterns and behaviors exist, and then try to change the person's relationship to those thoughts and behaviors (rather than relying on changing the thoughts and behaviors themselves). I believe it is helpful, as it focuses on coping and dealing with the situation. While the disease exists and creates the Lyme Brain, a therapy that depends on changing thoughts and behaviors may be an uphill battle. A therapy that helps the patient deal with the results of the disease process may be much more helpful. Cognitive-behavioral therapy works with the process at hand, helping the person find tools, coping strategies and adaptive behaviors, which can provide a great sense of empowerment and control.

ENERGY PSYCHOLOGY

Energy psychology is a field that encompasses a range of different techniques and approaches to break through blockages in emotions, cognition and health. It works with energy patterns and the bioenergetic field along with other more traditional therapeutic tools. It can quickly and effectively clear blockages and traumas, usually without having to dredge up past or painful feelings or experiences. It is truly a mind-body modality.

Energy psychology sessions might include elements of assessment through attunement and muscle testing, and strategies to affect change that might incorporate body postures, eye positioning or movement, tapping techniques on meridians or points, and other tools that work to balance the relationship between the bioenergetic systems of the body and cognitive-behavioral-emotional patterns. The premise is to rebalance the energetic systems of the body through interactions with biofields and meridians.

Energy psychology may seem a little more "out there" for some. However, I have experienced it personally and have seen how quickly and profoundly shifts occurred in my own life. Now I do not hesitate to recommend it to patients. I just encourage them to keep an open mind!

One example of a technique that falls under the umbrella of energy psychology is the Emotional Freedom Technique (EFT), also known as the tapping technique. EFT works on the meridians of the body, which requires tapping specific points in a certain order while voicing positive affirmations. The combination of these two elements helps to "short circuit" the emotional blockage and restore balance to the system.

What I love about EFT is that it is easy to learn and can be practiced in a few minutes a day as many times as needed and on any topic or issue. It can be used for everything from overcoming sugar cravings to deep traumas from past events. The results are instantaneous! I remember one day when I had to go to a location that I had not been to since a good friend of mine had had a gruesome accident and died there. I had traumatic memories of that event because I had been right there with him. I experienced severe anxiety whenever I thought about returning to that place, and yet I simply had to. I did a few minutes of tapping around the issue and the anxiety melted away. I still thought of him when driving to that place, but it was not traumatic. I was able to think of good memories, and although I did think of the last time I saw him there, it didn't trigger feelings of panic and trauma as it had before.

Dr. Mercola has a section on EFT on his website. Gary Craig, who is one of the developers of EFT, also has a book and a website (www.emofree.com). While there are plenty of skeptics, I have seen EFT bring profound changes in many individuals. Because it's a therapy that one can learn and practice at home in a short period of time (and for free), I believe it is worth checking out. For those who want professional guidance or want more advanced energy psychology work, there is a practitioner listing at www.energypsych.org.

Another therapy that falls under the umbrella of energy psychology is Psych-K. Remember when we talked about Bruce Lipton's work (*The Biology of Belief*) and epigenetics? He firmly believes that most limitations occur on the subconscious level, and subsequently, shifts must also occur on the subconscious level. However, while having this strong belief, he had not yet developed a strategy to address it. Then a psychotherapist named Rob Williams, M.A., developed and provided the program that addresses the limiting beliefs that occur on the subconscious level. This technique has gained popularity around the world as people find freedom from limitations. See www.psych-k.com for more information and a practitioner listing.

I believe that all of these psychological tools are valuable and have a lot to offer. In a nutshell, here's how I would guide my patients:

❖ Traditional counseling or psychotherapy—for those who are dealing with relational issues, feel unsupported or have high levels of stress.

❖ Cognitive-behavioral therapy—for those who need more help to figure out how to deal with their Lyme Brain responses on a day-to-day level (e.g., through healthier coping skills and adaptive behaviors).

❖ EFT—for those who would love a tool that they can use quickly and easily for a variety of purposes, including physical elements, such as pain and cravings, and emotional elements, such as anxiety and feeling overwhelmed; and for those who are self-motivated to learn it and practice it.

❖ Energy psychology—for those who have significant, deep-seated traumas or emotional issues to overcome, including PTSD.

❖ Psych-K—for those who feel that they live in negative/limiting beliefs such as "I'll never get well," "my situation is hopeless" or "I'll never be happy."

Some people can benefit from a combination of therapies, and they are not mutually exclusive. One's prominent situation as well as one's openness to energetic approaches to health will help guide what will be the best for any given individual.

CHAPTER 25

LYME DISEASE AND PTSD:

IS THERE AN ASSOCIATION?

———◦✕◦———

Robert Bransfield, M.D., a prominent Lyme expert and psychiatrist, presented information about post-traumatic stress disorder (PTSD) in Lyme patients at the ILADS annual conference in 2014. He rightly said that this is something that is rarely discussed, acknowledged or addressed. Yet PTSD can be incredibly painful and difficult to overcome, and so I love that this brilliant doctor is shedding some light on it based on what he has observed.

Dr. Bransfield sees a connection between Lyme disease and PTSD but acknowledges that some people have PTSD from events or traumas prior to, and separate from, their Lyme disease. He also sees that Lyme patients may be more susceptible to PTSD and that the experience of Lyme disease can actually cause PTSD in some individuals. He believes that infections make one more susceptible to PTSD via their creation of inflammatory markers and the impact of those on the brain.

Dr. Bransfield has observed the presence of intrusive symptoms, such as thoughts, images, emotions, sensory perceptions, the re-experiencing of traumas and even seizures, in such patients. Granted, intrusive symptoms can occur outside of PTSD, but when PTSD is present, it can make them worse. Intrusive symptoms are also a hallmark of obsessive-compulsive disorder, which can also be a part of Lyme symptomatology.

Intrusive symptoms are one manifestation of PTSD. Others include hyperarousal (constantly on guard), avoidance and numbing. People with PTSD easily go into fight-fright-or-flight mode. In fight mode, there is hyperarousal, and people can overreact to events and occurrences. There can also be avoidance in fight mode. In fright mode, there may be under arousal and psychic numbing, and people may freeze and underreact. In flight mode there can be avoidance. The result of all of these is a dysregulated stress response.

One of the features that Dr. Bransfield describes as the association between Lyme and PTSD is the elevation we see in Lyme patients of TNF-alpha, CRP, IL-6 and IL-1-beta. These are inflammatory markers that tend to predispose one to intrusive symptoms. There is increased activity of the amygdala, which is the part of the brain that directs emotional responses, and the hippocampus, which deals with factual content. The inflammatory cascade can mess with these areas of the brain and cause the disruption and lack of distinction between the two areas. In the PTSD process, an external or environmental cue leads to a traumatic memory association that leads to a re-experiencing of the initial event, which then leads to the fight-flight-or-fright response. That can be reflective of an overactive amygdala (leading to the focus on the emotional trauma) and a hippocampus that does not adequately support an awareness of the here and now. (The here and now might be completely safe, but the person with PTSD will not feel safe. They are trapped in the disturbed emotions.) Imaging supports this. Functional MRIs in PTSD tend to show an overactive amygdala and atrophy in the hippocampal regions. Dr. Bransfield also cites C-reactive protein, a blood marker of inflammation, as another marker of PTSD.

PTSD can be treated with various forms of therapy. Some people find various medications helpful. In the words of Dr. Bransfield himself, "Recovery is mastery over adversity."

SECTION 6:

THERAPIES TO HELP
LYME BRAIN

CHAPTER 26

NEUROFEEDBACK

———⊰✕⊱———

Neurofeedback is one of my favorite therapies, and I've seen it work wonders for Lyme Brain. I have had patients go from only sleeping two hours per night to sleeping full nights after a few sessions of neurofeedback. Others, after years of not feeling creative due to their Lyme disease, have started doing art again. Many others have reported significant gains in cognitive function after sessions of neurofeedback. It can also help with anxiety and depression.

Neurofeedback works to stabilize the frequency patterns of the brain. These are the brainwave patterns that are measured when one has an electroencephalogram (EEG). So far, we've talked about the *structure* of the brain, meaning the neurons with their axons and dendrites, and glial cells. We've talked about the *chemistry* of the brain with various neurotransmitters, and now, we are talking about the *electrical* activity of the brain.

Brainwave patterns can be classified as alpha, beta, delta, gamma and theta. Each grouping encompasses a particular range of frequencies, and each has its own characteristics.

For example, the alpha brainwave state is typically a relaxed state where one feels mindful and meditative. It is associated with increased creativity and a reduction in depression. Beta waves are heavily involved in cognitive functions; we are alert, focused, engaged and task-oriented. Delta and theta waves appear in the realm of sleep or very deep meditative states. Gamma waves are the fastest brainwaves and relate to the processing of information from different brain areas. They have been associated with higher states of conscious perception.

From these brief descriptions, we can see that one thing is clear. If you get stuck in one brainwave state or you have a dominance of a certain frequency range, it can impact your ability to function. If you have alpha dominance, you may feel dreamy or spacey, which could be a good thing or a bad thing depending on the context! Without sufficient beta waves, focusing or concentrating on anything will be challenging. Without the delta and theta waves, good quality, deep, restorative sleep could be elusive.

Many psychoemotional and psychological symptoms have some association with imbalances in brainwave activity.

Neurofeedback works to bring erratic brainwave patterns back into balance. First, it detects where waves are out of balance via electrodes on the head that measure brain frequency activity, much like an EEG. What happens from there depends on the fundamental principle of biofeedback: when the body is presented with information about its own functioning and given the encouragement and opportunity to change, it will do so. (This can also be done via heart rate, blood pressure, galvanic skin response and other means, but I am just talking about neurofeedback here, which in effect is biofeedback for the brain.)

The computer reads the brainwave activity and assesses where the imbalances are. The person receiving the therapy is listening to music, or in some neurofeedback systems, watching a video or playing games. When the brainwave patterns are healthy and balanced, the music plays uninterrupted. When the brainwave patterns are erratic, there are tiny breaks in the music that are barely perceptible to the ear (in the system I use, it sounds like very faint, brief scratches on an old record). The brain learns that it gets rewarded for operating within healthy frequency patterns and will start pulling itself into those patterns to continue the rewards.

Over a series of sessions, the brain is trained to operate in those healthy frequency patterns more frequently. I use the analogy of going to the gym and doing a bicep curl. If you go to the gym one time and lift a weight twenty times, your muscle will not be stronger by the next day (even though it might be sore!). However, if you go to the gym two or three times a week for several weeks, your muscle will be stronger, *even at rest*. You have trained a stronger muscle, and you can use that muscle more effectively in your everyday life. So it is with neurofeedback and the brain. After a series of sessions, the brain will operate in its newly learned, healthier pattern *all the time*, not just during the session. That means great things for your everyday functioning.

There are many different neurofeedback devices but all work on the same basic premise. In my practice, I utilize the Zengar NeurOptimal system, and I love it because instead of the practitioner setting the parameters of which bandwidths to upregulate and which to suppress, the machine assesses 16 different points and brings them all into balance simultaneously. Not only does this prevent any user error if the practitioner makes an incorrect assessment, but it also prevents any side effects or negative impacts. It is a gentle but deeply effective system, and I have seen tremendous benefits for Lyme Brain.

CHAPTER 27

HOME-BASED

BRAINWAVE ENTRAINMENT

—◦◦◦◦◦—

Neurofeedback is wonderful and would be my first choice, but there are also some alternatives for those for whom may not be able to get to a clinic for regular treatments or for those whom neurofeedback is not financially viable.

There are various systems that utilize brainwave entrainment in an audio format that one can do at home. Historically, they were based on the concept of the binaural beat (the formation of a third "sound" when one listens to two out-of-synch pure tone sine waves, one in each ear). In more recent generations, these technologies help to balance brain frequency activity using multiple harmonically layered frequencies to calm and balance brainwave patterns. These programs also work on whole brain synchronization, balancing left and right hemispheres.

HoloSync is one of the more popular home brain entrainment systems and one that I have used and liked myself. LifeFlow is another one that I have experienced (visit their website for a free demo). The one that I recommend the most is the Insight program. It is much less expensive and there are no other levels to purchase. Everything you need is on one CD. It is a 24-minute program that sounds like gentle rain to the user. It promotes relaxation, better sleep, less anxiety and pronounced relief from stress. They also have a Focus CD, which as the name suggests, is tailored to promote mental clarity, focus and concentration; that is an optional add-on to their primary program.

Another system I like is BrainTap Technologies. They have a library of thousands of guided meditations and targeted audio sessions. The premise is similar to the above-mentioned programs in that it aims to assist in retraining your brain in healthier patterns; however, these are tailored to more specific topics, such as pain management, greater clarity and healthy sleep habits. They also offer an optional headset with visual and audio entrainment.

Many meditators have used these systems to get to deeper levels of meditation. I know that for me, meditation in silence is a total no-go. However, I do find that sitting and listening to the rain is very easy. My to-do lists don't cycle through my mind as much as they might in a silent atmosphere!

Although I believe that professional-level neurofeedback is always going to provide the most beneficial therapeutic experience, in the absence of that, a relatively inexpensive and easy-to-use program such as Insight is definitely worth it. In less than half an hour per day, it can provide a calmer, more balanced mental state and improvements in memory, clarity, focus and concentration.

CHAPTER 28

HYPERBARIC OXYGEN THERAPY (HBOT)

———◇———

Hyperbaric oxygen therapy (HBOT) is a therapy that increases oxygenation of the body including the brain. It is a chamber or tank filled with 100% pure, pressurized oxygen in which one lies down or sits. The therapy is typically 90 minutes in duration, and there are different kinds of chambers. Some only fit one person (single-place chambers), while others look more like a room and can fit up to 20 individuals (multi-place chambers).

HBOT has long been used in allopathic medicine with a wide range of uses: burns; major infections; wound healing, including diabetic ulcers; strokes; blood chemistry changes, such as "the bends" (a result of too much nitrogen in the blood) in scuba diving; carbon monoxide poisoning; and radiation injury, to name just a few. HBOT chambers are widely used in hospital settings. However, sadly, Lyme disease is not on their approved list of conditions treated, leaving people to find private, independent clinics for this application. This can make the therapy quite expensive and cost-prohibitive for some. For others, it can be challenging to find a private clinic offering this therapy in a convenient location.

HBOT is so beneficial for neurological issues. Because what is being pumped into the chamber is pure oxygen and the pressure is several times higher than normal air pressure, the oxygen easily diffuses through the alveoli in the lungs and is absorbed into the body. The oxygen that is carried throughout your body can help to fight infection (bacteria such as Borrelia are anaerobic and do not thrive in an oxygen-rich environment), so it does help to overcome the pathogens themselves.

HBOT also promotes healing in areas of damage throughout the body. In areas of cell or tissue damage, the extra oxygen also stimulates the growth of new blood vessels, allowing better influx of nutrients to the cells. It also helps reduce inflammation, which is a major issue in chronic Lyme disease.

Perhaps most importantly, HBOT can significantly contribute to neurological healing and function.[1] Multiple studies have shown that it enhances the regeneration of axons (the long thread-like part of a nerve cell along which impulses are conducted).

It also increases growth factors and stem cells, which promote healing. The increase in vascularization in the brain through enhanced oxygenation also helps to improve the function of cells that may have lost function or become dormant due to blood stagnation, poor nutrition or the inflammatory process.

I have seen HBOT help people with many kinds of neurological issues, ranging from stroke to autism to Lyme disease. In my Lyme patients, it has made a significant impact on cognitive function. I have also seen it help with psychiatric and psychoemotional symptoms.

HBOT has multiple benefits. The increase in oxygenation in the body serves to reduce inflammation; it helps to overcome the infection itself by putting the bacteria in an environment in which they cannot thrive; it increases the production of growth factors and stem cells that help regenerate damaged cells and tissues; and it increases healing in the central nervous system by enhancing the repair and regeneration of axons, which are needed to transmit nerve impulses.

People often ask me about the difference between hard-shell HBOT chambers and soft-shell (aka mild) HBOT chambers, and there is quite a significant difference. Hard-shell chambers provide 100% oxygen at a high pressure, usually in the range of 2.0-2.8 atmospheres. Soft-shell chambers reach pressures of 1.0 to 1.5 atmospheres, nothing like the levels attained in the hard-shell ones. Also, in mild HBOT, 100% oxygen is not being pumped in; it is ambient air.

To be fair, I have heard anecdotal reports of patients who experienced some improvements in cognition and mental status following mild HBOT treatments. They usually report improvements in energy levels, too. It does make sense to me that any increase in oxygenation in the body could provide some benefit. Certainly, soft-shell chamber treatments are less expensive, and some people actually install the units in their homes. However, if my patients are interested in HBOT, I strongly encourage them to jump in and use the hard chambers. There is so much more evidence in favor of their efficacy. Granted, HBOT is very time and money intensive, so it is not possible for everyone, but for those who can take advantage of it, I have seen it make a significant contribution to healing their brain and improving their neurological issues, including improved cognition and regulated emotional states.

REFERENCES

[1] Nazario, J, and D P Kuffler. "Hyperbaric oxygen therapy and promoting neurological recovery following nerve trauma." *Undersea Hyperb Med* 38, no. 5 (September-October 2011): 345-66.

SECTION 7:

OTHER BARRIERS TO RECOVERY FROM LYME BRAIN

CHAPTER 29

INTRODUCTION

Of course, nothing with Lyme disease is simple. When trying to heal Lyme Brain, there are other facets that should be considered as possible contributing factors. This is going to be a very brief synopsis, as this could be another entire book, but I want to share a few things that I look at in conjunction with Lyme treatment itself.

- ❖ Heavy Metals

- ❖ Methylation Defects

- ❖ Adrenal Health

- ❖ Thyroid Health

- ❖ Mold Toxicity

- ❖ A Toxic Environment

CHAPTER 30

HEAVY METALS

⸻⸰⋈⋄⸰⸻

Toxic metals, such as mercury, lead, cadmium and aluminum, can easily build up in the body. They may first float around in the bloodstream, but then they will be absorbed into the body tissues where they lodge and can cause strife. Where they lodge determines the amount and type of strife they cause. For some, it may be in the connective tissue, such as joints and muscles, causing arthritic symptoms and pain. For others, it may be the cardiovascular system, contributing to heart disease. (Did you know that in some European countries, a patient presenting with blockage of coronary arteries will be detoxed of lead before there is any consideration of bypass surgery?) For other people, toxic metals can lodge in the neurological tissue—yes, the brain. This can cause cognitive decline, memory loss, problems with focus and concentration, word-finding difficulties and a generally foggy-brained feeling. Sound familiar?!

Where do these metals come from? Mercury can come from eating the wrong kinds of fish, from vaccines (including flu shots) and from air pollution (coal-burning power plants pump out mercury vapor every day). Lead might still be coming from old lead pipes, lead paint and, in very small quantities, from tap water, another good reason to drink filtered water.

Assessing heavy metal load is best done through a urine test. Yes, almost all labs offer blood testing for heavy metals, but here's the problem. Metals only stay in the bloodstream for an average of 6 to 8 weeks once they enter the body. After that, they are taken up into the tissues where they cause their strife. So, unless the exposure is recent, the blood levels will appear normal. Similarly, if one does a urine collection without a provoking agent, it may well also appear normal, because urine is simply a filtration of the blood.

Therefore, the method I use is a provoked urine test. I give a dose of DMSA, an agent that chelates heavy metals. A chelator is an agent that prods metals out of the tissues and shoves them back in the bloodstream where the kidneys and bowels can excrete them through the stool and urine. Chelation is akin to detoxing but is specific to toxic metals.

The DMSA causes a dump of metals. We collect urine for six hours following ingestion, and voila! We see metals coming out and can quantify them. I have run hundreds of these tests, and although it's not a perfect science and doesn't tell us exactly how much of these metals are left in the body, there is a definite correlation; the more metals that are dumped, the more there is in the body. Another way I know this is that when I retest my patients every two months throughout their treatment, I see the levels coming down on each test even though I'm giving them the same provoking dose. As their body stores go down, their levels on the provoked urine test do as well.

The only time I hesitate to do the provoked urine test is in patients who are so sensitive that the dump of metals might produce too much detox and make them feel really lousy. Then we either lower the dose of DMSA or embark on a gentle heavy metal detox protocol until they're strong enough to tolerate the test.

Much can be done to rid the body of heavy metals. I have some "slow and steady" protocols for very sick, highly sensitive patients and some "gung ho" protocols for patients who are quite functional and we think that toxic metals are the key factor holding them back. Protocols typically involve a combination of either DMSA or EDTA (sometimes both) along with detox helpers such as alpha-lipoic acid, glutathione and Dr. Nicola's Detox Support Formula; and binders that "escort" metals out of the bowels and prevent reabsorption such as Dr. Nicola's Fiber Plus, chlorella and activated charcoal.

CHAPTER 31

METHYLATION DEFECTS

———⟩⟨———

Methylation refers to the process of adding a methyl group to many chemical compounds in the body. The process of methylation influences biochemical pathways in the body that regulate many different functions and processes, among them detoxification, neurotransmitter production and immune function. The DNA needs methyl groups to create healthy RNA, which creates healthy proteins, tissues and cells.

Some people have genetic defects in their methylation pathways, which can impact their entire body. About 50% of the population has genetic variants of the MTHFR enzyme that causes them to have some difficulty resynthesizing methionine from homocysteine. That's fancy science-speak for "their methylation pathways are screwed up." Now don't panic. While genetics might indicate a predisposition, methylation defects can be corrected using the correct supplementation and lifestyle choices. This is the focus of epigenetics (epi means "on" or "above"). This goes above and beyond the basic genetic structure to how we can influence transcription to our body tissues.

There are tests to determine if you have defects in your methylation pathways. Large labs such as Labcorp and Quest will test the basic MTHFR genes to see if there are defects there. They report as negative, heterozygous (just one copy of the gene is mutated) or homozygous (both copies of the gene show mutations). Remember, we have two copies of all our genes, one from our mother and one from our father. A patient with homozygous mutations may have a greater susceptibility to certain health problems, where a heterozygous mutation is a milder version.

Some private labs such as 23 & Me do more extensive testing for different single nucleotide polymorphisms (SNPs) and look much more in depth at the genetic makeup of an individual. There are also some online services that provide inter-pretations of such reports. However, be warned. It's a lot of information and can be quite confusing to wade through.

Methylation is an emerging area in medicine. It's very important and, at the same time, very complex and confusing. But there are ways to simplify it and take a sensible approach. If there are any genetic defects showing on the lab testing, one can supplement with methylated B vitamins such as methyl-folate and methyl-B12. These can provide the body with more of the methyl groups needed to methylate the DNA and support healthier transcription. This can switch on detox, enable immune cells to function better, and increase the flow of healthy neurotransmitters, reducing depression and anxiety and allowing for better cognitive function. One must be careful though, because while some methylation support is a good thing, too much can make things even worse. As with so many treatment approaches it is advisable to start low in dosing and build up gradually.

CHAPTER 32

ADRENAL HEALTH

———✕———

The adrenals are the stress management centers of the body. They're so tiny—pea size—and sit upon the kidneys. But boy oh boy do they take the hit for everything going on in our bodies.

Any stressor on the body can impact adrenal function: physical stressors such as pain, inflammation, infection and lack of sleep; emotional stressors such as family dynamics, worry and financial burdens; nutritional stressors such as poor dietary choices; and even "good" stressors such as too much exercise. All of these things take their toll.

Given that many Lyme patients have been ill for many years, it makes sense that the adrenal glands can really be struggling. Adrenal fatigue can manifest in many ways, but the most common is profound, unrelenting exhaustion. Others include low immune function, poor sleep quality, inability to heal and poor detoxification. Adrenal fatigue also impacts the metabolism, leading to weight gain. But most importantly in this conversation, adrenal fatigue can cause foggy brain as well.

There are three stages in the chronic stress response. In the first stage, cortisol, our main adrenal hormone, is actually elevated. This is a compensatory mechanism and a quite normal one. Theoretically, when there's a stress on the body, the adrenals pump out more cortisol to help us deal with it. Think of a bear jumping out from behind the tree or, maybe more realistically for us, a near-miss car accident. Cortisol helps us to react and respond. This could potentially be life saving, but the system was designed for short-term stressors, not long prolonged ones such as chronic illness. When the stress is ongoing, the adrenals will try to continue to produce more cortisol, but over time, they will not be able to keep that up, and levels will fall…and fall…and fall, until eventually they're way below normal. This is Stage 3 adrenal exhaustion.

Once again, all labs offer cortisol testing, but many take just a single sample via bloodwork. This can provide some good information but has limitations. My favorite test is a saliva test because it measures four different samples—morning, noon, afternoon and night. This is better because some people have normal levels in the morning, but mid-afternoon levels have crashed (along with their energy). Some people are low in the morning but recover throughout the day. Some are low in the morning but elevated at night, which might provide insight into sleep problems.

There are lots of adrenal support nutrients and herbs. Vitamins C, B5 and B6 are very helpful, along with balancing herbs such as rhodiola and ashwaghanda. Adrenal hormone precursors, such as DHEA and pregnenolone, can provide building blocks that the body can use to produce more cortisol. Siberian and Korean ginseng can be a little more stimulating, and licorice root can help rebuild the adrenals when cortisol is really low. I prefer to use natural treatments taken over time to address adrenal fatigue, but in some patients where cortisol seems to have packed up and gone on vacation, I might use a little hydrocortisone to prop the body up until it returns. High cortisol, although less common, can benefit from those balancing herbs also, along with phosphatidylserine, a compound shown to lower excessive cortisol. High cortisol can drive anxiety and irritability, which can compound Lyme Brain problems.

CHAPTER 33

THYROID HEALTH

———⋊⋉———

The thyroid is a butterfly-shaped gland that sits across the neck. It produces the T4 hormone, which circulates around the body and is converted to T3, the active form of the thyroid hormone. The pituitary gland, which snuggles up under the brain, sends TSH to the thyroid to tell it to produce hormones, which then works on a reverse feedback loop. The lower the thyroid hormone levels are in the blood, the more TSH will be produced by the pituitary, because it is desperately trying to give instruction to the thyroid gland to up its production. Hence, when you see a high TSH level on labs, it actually reflects low thyroid function, and vice versa.

The thyroid regulates metabolism, amongst other things. Low thyroid function will make one very sluggish and fatigued, foggy-brained, constipated, depressed and a poor sleeper. It can produce dry skin, dry course hair, brittle nails, thinning eyebrows on the outer parts and a dull complexion. Many Lyme patients experience weight gain with their illness, and the thyroid may be partly to blame for this.

I often associate thyroid dysfunction with the co-infection Babesia. In fact, I associate most hormonal shenanigans with the co-infection Babesia. So this reiterates the point of treating all co-infections adequately, which can help hormones get back in line.

Given that most Lyme patients experience fatigue, poor sleep quality, night waking, depression and weight gain, looking closely at thyroid function makes sense. Unfortunately, many primary care doctors do a quick TSH check, and as long as it's in the broad range of 0.45–5, they consider everything normal and move on. There are two problems here. First, the ideal range of TSH is actually 0.45–2. Anything above 2 and I get suspicious of low thyroid function. Second, a TSH alone is not enough of an indicator. We at least need a free T3 and free T4, and preferably a reverse T3, to get a good picture. I also order the autoimmune thyroid markers—anti-TPO and anti-thyroglobulin—as many Lyme patients have autoimmune processes going on in their bodies, which can be assisted by compounds such as low dose naltrexone and a gluten-free diet. If T3 and T4 are low to normal and the clinical picture fits, I will consider supplementing with thyroid hormone. I've found that it makes a world of difference in many of my patients, especially in regard to energy and brain function.

The thyroid can be supported with natural supplements such as iodine, kelp, selenium and thyroid glandulars. There are also prescription "natural" thyroid medications like Armour and Nature-throid. Both of these are from a porcine source. My favorite by far is bio-identical, compounded T3 and T4 taken in a 1:4 ratio to mimic the body's natural production. Bio-identical means that it is produced to match the biochemical structure of human hormone exactly. It's not "natural" per se, because it is synthesized in the lab; however, because it matches our own thyroid hormone, the body can assimilate it much better (and the "natural" thyroid medications are only really natural if you're a pig, in my opinion, but that's neither here nor there!).

Thyroid supplementation that is started low and built up gradually until the right dose is attained can lead to more energy, a clearer brain, better quality sleep and a happier outlook. I have seen significant changes in cognition and mental alertness through correcting hormone imbalances, and if sleep can be improved with healthier thyroid function, that will further add to the mental benefits.

CHAPTER 34

MOLD TOXICITY

———◦∞◦———

Mold toxicity in the body can be another reason why some people struggle to recover from Lyme disease. In some ways, Lyme and mold toxicity have a lot in common. Both impact every system of the body, create toxicity in the body that is hard to recover from, have profound impacts on the neurological system and take advantage of genetic predispositions such as HLA phenotypes and methylation dysfunction.

The area of mold toxicity is a complex one. The expert on this topic is Dr. Ritchie Shoemaker, M.D., who has written an in-depth book called *Mold Warriors*. See his website www.survivingmold.com for more information.

Molds are types of fungi that can grow and reproduce to form spores. Mold grows indoors and outdoors, and is typically worse in damp environments. Some mold is visible, like the type we see growing on old food, but some is not. Black mold (Stachybotrys chartarum) is one of the most toxic types of mold. It is greenish-black in color and can grow indoors or outdoors.

Mold illness can be hard to test for directly. There are some labs that measure antibodies to various molds (we use US Biotek, but it's a very basic panel that only shows five different types of mold). The more effective way to assess the impact of molds on the body is to test a number of different markers including neurotoxic markers and inflammatory markers. Dr. Shoemaker uses the following lab markers as part of his assessment: VIP, melanocyte-stimulating hormone, TGF beta-1, C4a, HLA testing, anti-gliadin antibodies, ACTH/cortisol, VEGF, anticardiolipins, ADH, MMP-9 and leptin. If that all sounds quite complicated, it's because it is! Dr. Shoemaker also has a test on his website called a Visual Contrast Sensitivity (VCS) test that one can take online to assess the impact of mold on the neurological system. Real Time Labs offers a urine test that measures mycotoxins, and I find that test to be very helpful, too.

The first step in addressing mold issues in the body is to check, double-check and triple-check that there are no current exposures. There is no point in pursuing any further treatment options if there are sources of mycotoxins still entering the body. For some people, avoiding the source of exposure is enough to have them feeling better. The next step is the use of cholestyramine (CSM). This is a binder—its on-label use is for high cholesterol, as it binds fatty acids and helps to remove them from the body rather than allowing their absorption. But it can also bind neurotoxins, which helps mold patients significantly. It does have some downsides. It can produce constipation, and it needs to be taken three times daily on an empty stomach, which makes compliance quite difficult. But for those with mold toxicity, it's the most obvious treatment to try. Some may do better with activated charcoal and certain types of clays that act as more gentle binders.

Mold toxicity and Lyme disease together is a real double whammy. Definitely the comorbidities make recovery from each more challenging, but it can be done! If you suspect mold toxicity might be a factor in your case, Dr. Shoemaker's website is an excellent place to start gathering information. It also has a listing of practitioners who are certified in his protocol.

CHAPTER 35

A TOXIC ENVIRONMENT

Aside from molds, there are other sources of toxicity in your home. Cleaning products are the first that come to mind. Many of these products are laden with chemicals, some of which have very strong scents and can add to toxicity simply by breathing in their fumes. Skin contact with these products is another route of entry into the body. This may not seem like a big deal to a person who is not impacted by chronic illness, but for Lyme patients, every chemical exposure is significant.

There are many non-toxic cleaning products on the market. As demand for these products increases, more and more appear. I have numerous patients who have replaced their more toxic cleaning products one by one as they ran out, which spaced out the expense and made it less overwhelming. Ninety percent of my patients who have done this report feeling better when exposed to the new, non-toxic products. The Environmental Working Group is a great website for seeing how various natural products measure up, helping you to discern which ones are the most effective while being the least toxic (www.ewg.org).

Electromagnetic frequencies (EMFs) are another source of pollution. Those of us who live in cities are exposed to large amounts of EMFs—from Wi-Fi and cell phones to telecommunication towers and power lines. As much as we love all our wireless and Bluetooth devices, they are major sources of EMFs. So, are we all supposed to move out to the country to escape them? Not necessarily, and it's not like the rural areas are devoid of them either! What we can do is try to minimize their impact. Removing wireless devices in the bedroom is a great step. Many of my patients have reported that they slept better once they removed such things from their bedroom altogether. Using landline phones where possible rather than cell phones (and not the cordless ones either!), minimizing cell phone usage, having wired broadband Internet rather than Wi-Fi and avoiding Bluetooth devices—these things can all help. And it's worth it to avoid living in houses right near power lines.

There are various contraptions and devices on the market that are supposed to help reduce EMF radiation, such as earthing mats and sheets, EMF-protective clothing and protective cages. I find it hard to discern which of these are credible and which are not, so my first step is always to remove as many of the sources as possible. Since EMF pollution can't be felt right away, it is insidious and can be a major contributor to symptoms of Lyme Brain.

Another source of toxicity is through foods and water. In most areas, tap water contains traces of toxic metals such as lead and arsenic. It is also high in fluoride, a known neurotoxin, and chlorine. In fact, there are more than 80 "regulated" contaminants in our tap water, and even more unregulated toxins. Bottled water may be a better bet, but even then, research must be done to check the standards of individual brands. In many ways, I think a good water filtration system set up at the faucet is a better choice, and even better again is a whole house filtration system, because chemicals and toxins in water can access the body even by taking showers, brushing our teeth and so on.

Another source of toxins is through our food. Conventionally grown fruits and vegetables are laden with pesticides and fertilizers. Meat and poultry are reservoirs of antibiotics and hormones that are used to keep them disease-free and rapidly growing. Even farmed fish, which are typically fed grain, are more susceptible to heavy metals and other toxins, which change its healthy omega-3 fatty acids to less healthy ones. Eating organic produce and dairy, grass-fed beef and organic meats and poultry, and choosing wild-caught fish, will not only reduce your toxic intake of chemicals and pollutants, but will give you better quality food with higher nutrient levels.

— ✕ —

This is not an exhaustive list of contributors to Lyme Brain and barriers to recovery, so not all of them will apply to everyone. However, cleaning these areas can go a long way towards relieving the burden on your brain. Instead of feeling completely overwhelmed by these ideas, I suggest that you choose one or two things to ask your doctor about that haven't been covered in your treatment so far, and pick one or two things you can do at home to help yourself. Next month, reread the list and pick another one or two things. This way, progress will be made in a systematic way without being unrealistic or overwhelming.

SECTION 8:

PEDIATRIC CONSIDERATIONS

CHAPTER 36

LYME BRAIN IN CHILDREN

According to the Centers for Disease Control, 25% of Lyme disease cases are children. Children have three times the rate of other age groups, and the highest prevalence of Lyme is in boys aged 5-9.[1] Children love to be out in nature, cuddle pets and are low to the ground where ticks are.

Needless to say, we need to be highly cognizant of how Lyme disease impacts the neurological function of children; it just might not be the same as in adults. Children are also inherently tricky to assess: they may have limited language with which to describe what they are experiencing. They don't have as much "before" to compare with their "after" and neurological changes are an inherent, natural part of their lives, so it can be hard to say what is "normal" and what may be caused by an infectious illness such as Lyme disease. A good example is a child who struggles academically once they move from middle school to high school. This could be a sign of chronic illness holding them back, or it could be that the transition from middle school to upper school is difficult—bigger class sizes, new classmates and the loss of other friends to other schools can impact their experience.

Children with Lyme can manifest a host of different symptoms including headaches, chest pain, malaise, insomnia, joint pain and swelling, and so on. Most of the symptoms seen in adults can be also seen in children. However, since we are talking about Lyme Brain in this book, I will focus mostly on the behavioral and cognitive issues that arise.

In a 2013 presentation at the annual ILADS conference, Ann Corson, M.D. estimated that 90% of children have deterioration in school performance due to cognitive dysfunction secondary to Lyme disease. She cites some common issues as:

❖ Difficulty with concentration and attention

❖ Easy distractibility

❖ Often labeled as ADD/ADHD

❖ Word and name retrieval problems

❖ Short-term memory difficulties

❖ Decreased reading comprehension

❖ Impaired speech fluency

❖ Dyslexic-like errors

❖ Loss of mathematical skills

❖ Light/sound/visual overstimulation

The psychosocial aspects of this can be profound. Parents and teachers alike may assume that the child is simply daydreaming, not trying in school, creating symptoms to avoid going to school or avoiding homework. Parents can feel frustrated as their kids spend hours trying to do homework that they think with a little more focus could get done in half the time.

Teachers who do not have an understanding of Lyme and its impact may not provide the understanding and intellectual accommodations that the child needs. This can be heightened by the fact that the children often *look* normal. Educating the teachers and administrative staff of the school is so important and yet can be an uphill battle, especially in the realm of chronic Lyme disease, which is so controversial.

Children can feel isolated in their experience. Their friends are still running around, having fun and keeping up with school, and yet they know that they are falling behind. Their friends do not relate to them in the same way. At best, they may reject them, and at worst, ridicule or belittle them.

These issues can certainly shift the dynamics within the family as well. One sibling who gets a lot of attention for their health issues or their school/behavioral issues can result in the other one(s) feeling resentful and neglected. Sometimes parents are not on the same page about what is going on for their child and may be at odds as to the correct path for medical care or schooling. Sadly, I have seen marriages divide and dissolve more than once over children's health issues. The whole situation places a tremendous strain on the family unit as a whole.

There are a few key pieces that I think are so important to help children through:

❖ Ask for reasonable accommodations at school to help them cope until they are able to get back to their full load. This may be anything from shortening their school day, limiting their homework assignments, providing more time for them to complete tests or breaking up their work and tests into smaller units.

❖ Give a lot of encouragement at home, in particular, reinforcement that these challenges are a part of their illness; *this is not who they are*. While adults with Lyme Brain can at least rationally affirm to themselves that their deficits are caused by their illness and, as such, are temporary, children may simply feel stupid, inferior, worthless and overly frustrated.

❖ Seek out help and support to assist in coping with the situation, whether from a Lyme-literate psychotherapist, family therapist or even a coach. I have a teenage patient right now who is working with a coach to help her navigate her illness, which includes strategies to compensate for her cognitive and emotional deficits. It's making a world of difference for her and is giving her the confidence she needs to go off to college in a few weeks.

REFERENCES

[1] Centers for Disease Control and Prevention. *Lyme Disease Graphs*. 1995-2014. http://www.cdc.gov/lyme/stats/chartstables/incidencebyagesex.html (accessed September 15th, 2015).

CHAPTER 37

AUTISM AND LYME DISEASE

———⋈———

Rates of autism spectrum disorders (ASD) are reaching epidemic proportions. According to the CDC, autism now affects 1 in 68 children. ASD is five times more prevalent in boys: 1 in 42 boys are affected compared to 1 in 189 girls.[1]

Several years ago, the Lyme-Induced Autism Foundation was created to further research and education into the link between Lyme disease and ASD. Clearly, not all kids with ASD have Lyme disease; however, there is some overlap between the two. Clinicians that were polled by that organization reported that their ASD patients who tested positive for Lyme ranged from 20% all the way up to 90%. The results indicated that there was some overlap, but further research is definitely needed.

I work with quite a few kids who have both diagnoses. Of course, association does not imply causation, but it is not out of the question to think that Lyme disease and its neurological manifestations could cause a child to present with ASD. Perhaps, too, the genetic methylation pathway defects that make one more susceptible to neurotoxic stress from Lyme also render one more susceptible to autism because of the difficulty in detoxifying heavy metals such as mercury, and through dysregulation of the immune system, disruption of neurotransmitter production and the general inability to detoxify.

One of the challenges with this group is that they have very sensitive systems and often have dysbiosis of the gut. This means that antibiotic therapies can be hard for them to tolerate and, many times, will make their gut dysbiosis so bad that it creates more of the ASD symptoms. Therefore, herbal treatments and essential oils may be better options for ASD children than antibiotics themselves. I have used our own RestorMedicine herbs as well as Byron White Formulas, essential oils and a variety of supplements in children with good results. Antifungal therapy is typically warranted, and I find nystatin is a great help along with liposomal

Biocidin (a herbal formula by BioBotanical). Detoxification may be even more important in children than adults, so that should be prioritized.

REFERENCES

[1] Centers for Disease Control and Prevention. *Autism Spectrum Disorder (ASD) Data & Statistics.* 2000-2010. http://www.cdc.gov/ncbddd/autism/data.html.

CHAPTER 38

MENTAL ILLNESS AND LYME DISEASE

———◆———

Psychiatric involvement is another aspect of Lyme Brain to be conscious of in children.

Mental illness, in general, is a huge problem in children and adolescents. Anyone in the United States can attest to the gravity of the problem by observing some of the mass shootings and suicides that have occurred in the past five years. In the United States alone, 4,000,000 children and adolescents suffer from a serious mental disorder that interferes with functioning. In fact, one-half of all lifetime mental disorders start by age 14.[1] I am not implying that Lyme disease is the root cause of this mental illness, but it is important to consider tick-borne illness as a possible cause.

Children with Lyme disease have exhibited psychiatric symptoms such as rages, social withdrawal, suicidal ideation (approximately 40% of kids, according to parents, with 11% actually making a suicide attempt or gesture), irritability and mood swings, anxiety, panic attacks, paranoia, hallucinations and, in some cases, violent and criminal behavior. Children can also have violent and vivid dreams that are frightening and disturbing for them.

Rosalie Greenberg, M.D., a pediatric and adolescent psychiatrist, presented on tick-borne illness and the pediatric brain at the ILADS convention in Washington, DC in 2014. She described her work with children who are diagnosed with bipolar disorder (she has also written a book on the topic called *Bipolar Kids: Helping Your Child Find Calm in the Mood Storm*). Dr. Greenberg cites a study that she undertook of 14 subjects.[2] Of the 14, 6 were diagnosed with Mycoplasma, 3 with Borrelia, 10 with Babesia, and 4 with Bartonella. All 14 bipolar children were diagnosed with a tick-borne illness of some kind, with Babesia cited as the most common infection. However, only one of those children also presented with joint pain. This indicates that children may present differently than adults, and it also supports the idea that children tend to present with more central nervous problems than peripheral problems.

In another study of 11 children with anxiety and/or mood disorders, five males and six females between 6 and 13 years of age were examined.[3] Ten out of eleven children tested positive for a tick-borne illness (Fry lab testing was also performed and all 11 children tested positive on their tests). Four tested positive for Borrelia, eight for Babesia, one for Bartonella, two for Protomyxzoa and six for Mycoplasma pneumonia.

Therefore, in the two previous studies, of the 25 children diagnosed either as bipolar or having an anxiety/mood disorder, 12 had Mycoplasma pneumonia, 7 Borrelia, 17 Babesia and 5 Bartonella.

I also found it interesting that Babesia was easily the most common co-infection, where I have historically associated Bartonella with more severe psychiatric manifestations. This has significant clinical repercussions, and it reflects the importance of screening for all co-infections through lab work but also through observation and clinical presentation.

Certainly these studies are small and, as Dr. Greenberg herself stressed, need replication and further investigation. However, it does point to an association between tick-borne illness and psychiatric manifestations in children.

In conclusion, children have Lyme Brain, too, even though it may impact them somewhat differently than adults. Their natural rapid growth rate and developmental stages may make it hard to discern what could be abnormal and caused by chronic infection.

Children need a lot of support during this time, as they are sensitive to being different, standing out, or not keeping up with their peers. They will see their friends going off to play or participate in sports, or even go to the movies, but their symptoms may not allow them to do those things, so they will feel left out, which may lead to resentment. Sibling relationships can become strained and the unwell child will need more attention from the parents. Marriages can also become strained with the stresses of having a chronically ill child—everything from agreeing on the best treatment plan to financing often hefty medical bills.

I strongly believe that family therapy can be very helpful in navigating these complexities and giving children adequate support and space to process their illness.

Making appropriate accommodations while giving children as much of a semblance of normal life as possible is important.

For further reading on navigating Lyme disease with children, I highly recommend Sandy Berenbaum, L.C.S.W. and Dorothy Kupcha Leland's book *When Your Child Has Lyme Disease: A Parent's Survival Guide.*

REFERENCES

[1] Kessler, R C, W T Chiu, O Demler, K R Merikangas, and E E Walters. "Prevalence, severity, and comorbidity of 12-month DSM-IV disorders in the National Comorbidity Survey Replication." *Arch Gen Psychiatry* 62, no. 6 (July 2005): 617-27.

[2] Greenberg, Rosalie. "Tick-Borne Diseases and the Brain: Implications for Pediatric Psychiatry." *ILADS Conference 2014.* Washington, DC, October 10th, 2014.

[3] Greenberg, Rosalie. "Tick-Borne Diseases."

SECTION 9:

PUTTING IT ALL TOGETHER

CHAPTER 39

PRODUCTS AND PROTOCOLS

———⊰✕⊱———

Following are a few of my favorite products that incorporate many of the herbs and supplements that we discussed in the Natural Treatments section. Please remember that everyone is unique and has a different level of sensitivity. The doses recommended here are average doses. As always, if you are sensitive, you might dose much lower, and in general, we recommend starting low and building up gradually. I also recommend starting one new product at a time and staggering additions by at least a few days so that you can gauge how you feel on each one. Just to get started, I have summarized in table format the different herbs and nutrients we discussed in the Natural Treatments section so that you can see which individual ingredient offers which benefit(s). In the following pages, you will find product recommendations that combine these ingredients well and, finally, a summary of a typical dosing schedule.

First, let's recap our individual herbs and nutrients and their activities:

Product Name	Antimicrobial	Anti-inflammatory	Antioxidant	N
Garlic	•			
Andrographis	•	•		•
Polygonum	•	•	•	•
Cat's Claw	•	•		•
Teasel Root	•	•		
Olive Leaf	•	•	•	•
Artemisinin	•	•		
Cryptolepis	•			
Houttuynia	•			
Curcumin		•	•	•
Boswellia		•		•
Stephania		•		•
Proteolytic Enzymes		•		
Glutathione			•	•
Smilax Glabrae	•	•		
Pimpinella Anise		•		•
Molybdenum				
Yucca		•	•	
5-HTP				
Tyrosine				
GABA				
Phosphatidylcholine				
Phosphatidylserine				
Vinpocetine		•	•	•
Huperzine A				•
Lithuim				•
Vitamin B12				•
Resveratrol			•	
Acetyl-L-Carnitine			•	•
Alpha-Lipoic Acid		•	•	•
Omega-3 Fatty Acid		•	•	•
Lion's Mane Mushroom				•
Progesterone		•		•

tective	Neuroregenerative	Assist Detoxification	Balance Neurotransmitters	Cognitive Enhancers
		•		
	•	•		
			•	•
			•	
		•	•	
		•		
		•		
		•		
		•		
			•	
			•	
			•	
			•	
			•	•
				•
	•		•	•
	•	•	•	
	•	•		•
				•
	•	•	•	•
	•	•		
	•	•		
	•			•
	•			•

Here are some formulas and products that I love, that I think combine the ingredients we're looking for to help Lyme Brain, without having to take a hundred different things!

ANTIMICROBIALS

➢ Dr. Nicola's Lyme Support Formula (RestorMedicine) – tincture – 10 drops twice daily.
  - Guaiacum
  - Cat's Claw
  - Olive Leaf Extract
  - Andrographis
  - Japanese Knotweed

➢ Dr. Nicola's Teasel Root (RestorMedicine) – tincture – 5-10 drops twice daily.

➢ Dr. Nicola's Fresh Garlic (RestorMedicine) – tincture – 1-2 drops twice daily.

➢ Artemisinin SOD (Researched Nutritionals) – 100mg – 2 twice daily, or 2 three times daily, 4 days on/3 days off.

➢ HH2 Formula (Zhang) – capsules – 1 three times daily.

➢ Liposomal Biocidin (Bio-Botanical) – tincture – 1-3 pumps twice daily.
  - Bilberry, Noni, Milk thistle, Echinacea, Goldenseal, White willow, Garlic, Grapeseed extract, Black walnut, Raspberry, Fumitory, Gentian, Tea tree oil, Galbanum oil, Lavender oil, Oregano oil

  Note: Liposomal Biocidin is a great anti-fungal formula, as well as having activity against Borrelia and co-infections. It is particularly good for Lyme Brain as the liposomal form crosses the blood-brain barrier so well.

Byron White Formulas (Byron White)

➢ A-L Complex – tincture – 1-10 drops twice daily.

  - Allium sepa, Allium sativa, Juglans nigra, Armoracia rusticana, Zinziber officinale, Smilax officinalis, Syzygium aromaticum, Coptis chinensis, Gardinia jasminoidis, Musa paradisiaca, Artemesia annua, Citrus lemon, Astragalus membranaceous, Usnea barbata.

➢ A-BAB – tincture – 1-10 drops twice daily.
  • Azadlrachta indica, Curcuma xanthorrhiza, Uncaria tomentosa, Morinda officinalis, Uncaria rhynchophylla, Achillea millefollum, Blumea balsamifera.

➢ A-BART – tincture – 1-10 drops twice daily.
  • Allium sativum, Unacarla rhychophylla, Glycyrrhiza glabra, Azadlrachta indica, Citrus paradisi, Hemidesmus indicus, Syzygium aromaticum, Usnea barbata, Phytolacca americana.

DETOXIFICATION HELPERS

➢ Dr. Nicola's Smilax Glabrae (RestorMedicine) – tincture – 10-30 drops twice daily.

➢ Liposomal Glutathione (Researched Nutritionals) – liquid – 1 teaspoon first thing in the morning on an empty stomach.

➢ Dr. Nicola's Detox Support Formula #1(RestorMedicine) – tincture – 30 drops twice daily.
  • Astragalus
  • Burdock
  • Dandelion root
  • Goji berry
  • Lemon balm
  • Milk thistle
  • Wu-Wei-Zi fruit
  • Thorowax
  • Oregon grape root
  • Licorice root

➢ Dr. Nicola's Detox Support Formula #2 (RestorMedicine) – tincture – 30 drops twice daily.
  • Astragalus
  • Burdock
  • Dandelion root
  • Goji berry
  • Lemon balm
  • Wu-Wei-Zi fruit
  • Thorowax
  • Oregon grape root
  • Licorice root

➢ Molybdenum (Douglas Labs) – capsules – 500mcg – 1-2 daily.

ANTI-INFLAMMATORIES

➢ Dr. Nicola's Anti-inflammatory Formula (RestorMedicine) – tincture – 30 drops twice daily.
  • Boswellia
  • Holy basil
  • Curcumin (fresh turmeric)
  • Stephania
  • White willow

➢ CytoQuell (Researched Nutritionals) – capsules – 1 three times daily.
  • Black tea extract (decaffeinated)
  • N-Acetyl-L-Cysteine
  • Tumeric
  • Tocotrienols
  • Resveratrol

➢ InflaQuell (Researched Nutritionals) – capsules – 3 twice daily between meals.
  • Protease
  • Bromelain
  • Serrazimes
  • Papain

➢ Restore For Gut Health (Biomic Sciences) – liquid – 1 teaspoon three times daily before meals.
  • Lignite extracts 5mg
  • Trace minerals
  Note: I have been using Restore For Gut Health to help heal leaky gut and rebalance the gut microbiome. Many patients have not only found benefit for their digestion, but also for their cognitive function too.

BRAIN/COGNITION SUPPORT

➢ Dr. Nicola's Brain Support Formula (RestorMedicine) – tincture – 30-60 drops twice daily.
  • Lion's mane
  • Anise (pimpinella)

- Vinca minor (periwinkle)
- Gotu kola
- Ginkgo

➢ Cognicare (Researched Nutritionals) – capsules – 2 twice daily.
  - Vitamin B6 10mg
  - Vitamin B12 (methylcobalamin) 2500mcg
  - L-glutamine
  - L-tyrosine
  - Phosphatidylserine
  - Huperzine A 650mg
  - Acetyl-L-carnitine
  - Vinpocetine 780mg

➢ Omega-3 Plus (Researched Nutritionals) – capsules – 1000mg – 2 daily.

➢ Frankincense essential oil – 2-3 drops under the tongue twice daily.

➢ Lithium Orotate (Pure Encapsulations) – capsules – 5mg – 1-2 daily.

NEUROTRANSMITTER SUPPORT

➢ 5-HTP Synergy (Designs for Health) – capsules – 50mg – 1-2 twice daily between meals.

➢ Tyrosine (Pure Encapsulations) – capsules – 500mg – 1-2 twice daily between meals.

➢ Phenitropic (Biotics) – capsules – 300mg (as phenibut) – 1 twice daily.

➢ Neurolink (Designs for Health) – capsules – up to 3 twice daily.
  - Vitamin B6 (as Pyridoxal-5-Phosphate) 30 mg
  - L-Tyrosine 1200 mg
  - GABA 750 mg
  - L-Glutamine 600 mg
  - Inositol 600 mg
  - L-Taurine 600 mg
  - 5-HTP 150 mg

➢ Synaptamine (La Vida RDS) – liquid – ½ ounce twice daily.

Proprietary blend of:-
- Pyridoxal-5-Phosphate
- Tyrosine
- L-Glutamine
- Rhodiola
- Griffonia seed
- 5-HTP
- L-Phenylalanine
- Chromium
- Passion Flower
- N-Acetyl-Cysteine
- Glucosamine N-Acetyl
- Arabinogalactan Fiber
- Aloe Vera Powder
- White Birch Bark
- Boswellia Serrata
- Spirulina

Note: this is a formula that supports a range of different neurotransmitters, especially the dopamine pathway. It has great application in situations of addiction and drug withdrawal, but has also worked well for generalized anxiety and depression, including that caused by tick-borne illness.

Where to purchase products:

RestorMedicine – Researched Nutritionals – Biotics – Restore For Gut Health – Synaptamine

www.shop.restormedicine.com

Designs for Health – Pure Encapsulations – Douglas Labs

www.emersonecologics.com (use access code 200772)

Byron White Formulas

www.byronwhiteformulas.com or call RestorMedicine to order 619 546 4065

DOSING SUMMARY

ANTIMICROBIALS

Dr. Nicola's Lyme Support Formula	10-20 drops twice daily
Dr. Nicola's Teasel Root	5-10 drops twice daily
Dr. Nicola's Fresh Garlic	1-2 drops twice daily
Artemisinin SOD	2 capsules twice daily, or 2 capsules three times daily, 4 days on/3 days off
HH2 Formula	1 capsule three times daily
Liposomal Biocidin	1-2 pumps twice daily
BWF A-L Complex	1-10 drops twice daily
BWF A-BAB	1-10 drops twice daily
BWF A-BART	1-10 drops twice daily

DETOXIFICATION HELPERS

Dr. Nicola's Smilax Glabrae	10-30 drops twice daily
Liposomal Glutathione	1 teaspoon daily
Dr. Nicola's Detox Support #1	30 drops twice daily
Dr. Nicola's Detox Support #2	30 drops twice daily
Molybdenum	1-2 capsules daily

ANTI-INFLAMMATORIES

Dr. Nicola's Anti-inflammatory Formula	30 drops twice daily
CytoQuell	1 capsule three times daily
InflaQuell	3 capsules twice daily between meals
Restore For Gut Health	1 teaspoon three times daily before meals

BRAIN/COGNITION SUPPORT

Dr. Nicola's Brain Support Formula	30-60 drops twice daily
Cognicare	2 capsules twice daily
Omega-3 Plus	2 capsules daily
Frankincense	2-3 drops twice daily
Lithium Orotate	1-2 capsules daily

NEUROTRANSMITTER SUPPORT

5-HTP	1-2 capsules twice daily between meals
Tyrosine	1-2 capsules twice daily between meals
Phenitropic	1 capsule twice daily
Neurolink	1-3 capsules twice daily
Synaptamine	½ ounce twice daily

SECTION 10:

INTERVIEWS

CHAPTER 40

INTRODUCTION

———✦———

In looking into any topic or area of study, especially one as diverse and complex as Lyme disease, I always think it is important to gather a range of opinions and perspectives. The following interviews will provide you with that. Two of the interviews are with patients who have been dealing with Lyme for many years and who have also researched and written extensively on the subject, giving them each a wealth of knowledge. Three of these interviews are with medical and allied health practitioners. Every one of them has such great knowledge, wisdom and experience to share.

CHAPTER 41

SCOTT FORSGREN

———⊶⊷⊶———

Scott, how long have you been recovering from Lyme disease?

I was diagnosed eight years into my illness, but I've been working on recovering my health for almost 20 years now. I had a tick bite in 1996, but my health really fell apart in 1997.

Did you experience Lyme Brain, and how did that manifest for you? How did it impact your life?

I definitely did. At my worst, I couldn't remember my home phone number or where I parked my car. I remember once when I was at work—we had three five-story parking structures, and I needed to get the security people to drive me around until I found my car. At one point, I had to live with my parents for a couple of months for the extra help, but I was fortunately able to contin- ue working. Thankfully, I had an understanding boss and I could amend my hours and work structure to fit my needs. For me, it was really important to use coping skills, like putting reminders on my phone and creating lists; I am a master at lists.

Today, fortunately, my cognitive skills are very good. It's important for people to re- member that their brain is still in there; the fog is just a layer on top of it. I've seen people time and time again react with extreme excitement when their treatment leads them to a glimpse of the way their brain used to work.

What were the therapies that you found most helpful?

The most important thing for me was detoxification, especially ammonia, which is common in Lyme, mycotoxins and aldehydes. Heavy metals also need to be con- sidered and addressed in order to minimize the impact of toxins on our cognitive functioning. I did lots of coffee enemas, which helped somewhat with brain clarity but helped a tremendous amount with pain and inflammation.

I like the Neuro-Antitox II formulas from Jernigan Nutraceuticals, especially for ammonia and neurotoxins/biotoxins. I did whatever else I could to help with detox such as infrared saunas, Biomat, ionic footbaths, homeopathic drainage remedies and numerous other options. For me, detoxification has always been my primary weakness and primary area of treatment focus.

It is important to note, though, that some of these toxins come from infections. For example, Candida may produce aldehydes and many other toxins. Parasites and Borrelia may produce ammonia. Thus, there is an aspect of detoxification that needs to focus on the source of the toxins and minimize that as well. Some toxins come from outside of us, but many of them come from inside.

Beyond that, some of the infections can directly impact our cognitive functioning as well. Thus, a holistic approach is needed that considers both toxic and infectious burdens.

What medications did you find most helpful?

For me, antibiotics helped overall with the nervous system symptoms but not as much with my brain. I had the experience of my nervous system being on fire, with a lot of burning symptoms. Antibiotics helped with that. I don't really remember any moments where I thought that the antibiotics were helping my brain come back. Having said that, I know people where Rocephin or other antibiotics did help a lot. It's been eight years since I took any antibiotics.

I never tried Provigil or any of the cognition meds. I did take cholestyramine to reduce toxins, and that helped quite a bit. I had tried antidepressants at one point along the way, but they were not helpful. I only stayed on them a few weeks, and they actually made me feel even more tired than I already did. Of course, that was back in the day when my illness was all in my head and no one took me seriously.

I think it's important to combine antimicrobial and detox elements. I'm not completely sure if it was the bug itself or the toxins from the bugs that contributed to most of my brain fog; it was likely a combination of both. I do think there are aspects of infection itself that impact the brain. There is research that shows infections in the brain of Alzheimer's patients, so we know that can play a partial role. Co-infections are also important to look at; they can play with our brains in terms of brain fog, anxiety, worrying, depression and OCD. Both Bartonella and Babesia, co-infections of Lyme, can result in a lot of mental and emotional symptoms.

Heavy metals also create a lot of brain fog. Mold, too. I know I lived in a moldy environment. It's hard to think clearly when you're exposed to poisons every day. But then, is the environment we're living in generally conducive with the brain being in top form? EMFs for example impact the brain directly and indirectly.

Then there are the obvious things like not drinking enough water and not pooping enough.

You mentioned the Neuro-Antitox formulas. What other supplements did you find most helpful?

Most of the supplements I like best involve detox and inflammation.

I like Takesumi Supreme by Supreme Nutrition products. I'll take that before times when I need to be "on." For the inflammatory piece, I'll use Beyond Balance Cyflacalm II. I find it good for inflammation in the nervous system. If I feel really toxic, I've used liposomal glutathione, and I often fall back to the coffee enemas to ramp up my detox.

To be honest, I've been a bit disappointed with some of the anti-inflammatory products—I always found coffee enemas to be better. For ammonia I have used zeolites, Neuro-Antitox II, butyrate, and other detox agents. I've used molybdenum for sulphur and have also read that it can help with aldehydes from Candida. I also use a lot of healthy fats such as MCT oil, coconut oil, and BodyBio Balance Oil and Phosphatidylcholine.

I have also just recently started exploring a product from Results RNA called ACN Neuro and think it warrants a mention in a discussion about brain and cognitive health. I'm pretty excited about its possibilities.

Did you find that your diet impacted your brain function? How?

I can't directly correlate brain function with diet, but I did adjust my diet to help reduce overall inflammation. I have been gluten free for a long time, which definitely helps to reduce inflammation. More inflammation is going to make brain function deteriorate.

I think it is important to be gluten free, to reduce or eliminate cow dairy, soy, nightshades, and anything else that we are known to be allergic to. Not eliminating food toxins makes it very difficult to make overall progress with our treatment protocol.

It's also important to reduce sugar. Sugar will feed Candida, which creates brain fog, too.

What lifestyle factors do you think are the most important?

Sleep is absolutely critical. Fortunately, that wasn't a major issue for me; I do well with melatonin, which also greatly helps the brain. I get 8–9 hours of sleep a night. If I get any less than that, I won't be sharp the next day. More recently, my primary mentor, Dr. Dietrich Klinghardt, has suggested liposomal melatonin may help detoxify the brain. No wonder I have loved it all these years!

I believe if people aren't sleeping well, that needs to be at the top of the list. Not sleeping well and not pooping well, they both need to be the top two priorities.

I probably also do less exercise than I need to. I do cycle regularly, though, and I find that it really helps me. If I'm having any flare-up of inflammation, I won't exercise during those times. Fortunately, I recently identified a source of ongoing mold exposure that was keeping me more inflamed, and since removing myself from that environment, the inflammation has definitely improved.

Which Lyme Brain therapies were you able to do at home on your own and which required the help of a doctor?

I did most of the detox stuff at home, like the coffee enemas. I used doctors to facilitate things like ordering tests for new information—energetic testing was important for me.

I did a few things on the pharmaceutical side such as low dose naltrexone. I did also spend several years on antibiotics. They certainly helped quite a lot the first year. I had quite a reduction in symptoms, but I'm not sure they helped that much after that. I think I'm still dealing with the Candida that resulted from the antibiotics. Additionally, I did them for so long because ten years ago, that was the only real option. Now, we have so many options that my path would have been very different and much more natural. I guess I'm grateful for having made progress using the antibiotics while also regretting having used them for so long.

Do you have any words of advice to Lyme patients with regards to Lyme Brain?

I would focus on the fact that there is hope for recovery. People who've been in a place where you are currently are now doing well and are having a happy, productive life. It's easy to forget that that possibility is still there.

I'm surprised at how many people don't know much about detox, or their doctors never talk about it and how to get stuff out. Much of my cognitive function comes back to how toxic I am on any given day.

Be hopeful and be optimistic!

Scott Forsgren is a blogger, health writer, advocate, and coach. He is the editor and founder of BetterHealthGuy.com, where he shares his 20-year journey through the world of Lyme disease, mold illness, and the myriad of factors that it often entails.

He has been interviewed on Lyme Ninja Radio, Lyme Less Live More, Essential Medcast, Beyond Wellness Radio, and Shift Series Interviews. He has been a speaker at the Autism Recovery Telesummit, Chronic Lyme Disease Summit, and Chronic Wellness Summit.

He has lectured on his recovery from chronic illness as an invited speaker of the Klinghardt Academy and at AutismOne. He has been fortunate to have written for publications such as Townsend Letter, Public Health Alert, Explore! and others.

He serves on the Board of Directors of LymeLight Foundation, which provides treatment grants to children and young adults dealing with Lyme disease. Today, Scott is grateful for his current state of health and all that he has learned on this life-changing journey.

CHAPTER 42

CONNIE STRASHEIM

Did you experience Lyme Brain, and how did that manifest for you?

Lyme Brain was certainly a problem for me. There were days when writing was really a struggle, and I had to just lie down and rest. I know that Lyme Brain is a big problem for many Lyme sufferers.

What were the therapies that you found most helpful?

I used phosphatidylcholine to increase levels of acetylcholine in my brain, which in turn helped to mitigate symptoms of brain fog. Phosphatidylcholine also helps to rebuild cell membranes and to detoxify the body. I also took a lot of omega-3 EFAs. I think it's important to measure cholesterol, too—if our healthy cholesterol is too low, we can't make steroid hormones, which then impacts our adrenal function and reproductive hormones.

I used bio-identical hormones to support adrenal and thyroid function, specifically pregnenolone, DHEA, progesterone and tri-iodo-thyronine, or T3. Bio-identical hormones can support the overall health of the body and provide energy, stamina, mood and cognitive support while healing from Lyme infections.

I also like amino acid therapy for restoring cognitive and other functions of the brain and body, but people need to be careful, as using single amino acids without getting lab tests done to determine what the body needs can cause further imbalances. For example, serotonin and dopamine both need to be present in the body in a certain ratio, or symptoms can worsen. If people have methylation defects, they may not utilize amino acids properly, which means that they won't be able to properly synthesize neurotransmitters.

At first, when I took amino acids, I got worse and had more brain fog, depression and fatigue. Once I began taking methylation supplements, I could slowly build up and take different combinations of amino acids to support my cognitive abilities and mood. I found L-tyrosine and 5-HTP to be particularly helpful. A few of the methylators that I used included methyl-B12, methyl-folate, P5P and SAM-e, based on my amino acid profile and methylation test results.

I think my healing was accelerated because of taking care of those aspects of my recovery. The amino acid therapy was great because it provided the raw materials to build the neurotransmitters. It took time—about eight months—but it made an amazing difference. But again, I don't recommend experimenting with amino acids on your own. You'll want to see a doctor and do lab testing to determine what you need. The same is true with bio-identical hormones.

I also did some neurofeedback training using a device called the Neurointegrator (from Clear Mind). This device helps to adjust brain wave activity and can be used to treat a variety of neurological conditions, including depression, anxiety, poor cognition and insomnia. The device comes with colored glasses that are used as part of the biofeedback program and help to regulate different brain functions. For example, yellow helps with anxiety, green helps with depression and blue helps with sleep. It modulates brain waves over time. The device is used a lot in kids with ADD and autism. It cost about $3200 for an at-home unit. There might be other neurofeedback devices around that aren't as pricey—different kinds of sound and light machines, for example.

What medications did you find most helpful?

Amitriptyline mitigated my symptoms for a period of time but, in the end, was damaging to my neurological system. It depleted my serotonin and exacerbated the very symptoms it was intended to treat. Benzodiazepines helped me to sleep for months during Lyme disease treatment but produced severe withdrawal symptoms and memory loss, which I am still struggling to recover from to this day. If I knew back then what I know now about antidepressants and sedative drugs, I would have never taken them, as they are extremely damaging to the body. I have found amino acid and hormone therapy, when properly dosed and taken along with other nutrients, to be far better for treating brain fog, insomnia and other neurological symptoms.

Did you find that your diet impacted your brain function?

Any food allergens create inflammation in the body, which can, in turn, impact cognitive functioning.

I think gluten is the main offender, and also most dairy products. As far as dairy products go, I have been able to eat some healthy organic cheese or a little bit of yoghurt, but that's it. I avoid soy and corn because they are genetically modified and common allergens. Bread itself isn't unhealthy, but rather, it's what has been done to it that's a problem. It's genetically modified and contains copious amounts of gluten, which damages the gut. When the gut is healthy, then the brain is healthy.

I do best on a diet of healthy organic animal protein, low glycemic fruits, veggies and nuts. Juicing greens also helped my brain and gut to function better.

What other factors made a big difference for you?

Healing my brain and body from the effects of depression. If people are dealing with depression, that will also affect mental and cognitive function, because depression often causes brain fog and an inability to concentrate.

Exercise also helped me. I found that if I walked for 45 minutes before I did intense work, this oxygenated my brain and I could work more effectively.

Prayer has also played a big role in restoring my cognitive function. My brain fog was usually worse in the morning, so I would spend most of my mornings in prayer and meditation, and would save more intense activity and writing work for the afternoon. It's important to fit your life around your energy patterns and do things when you function best.

I definitely think that toxins in the brain can also cause brain fog, and I found that doing coffee enemas and liver cleanses were beneficial. Liver and gastrointestinal function impact brain function and vice versa. I also found that coffee enemas could relieve feelings of anger and irritation.

Taking toxin binders for ammonia in the brain and other neurotoxins can also be helpful, as can looking for any causes of inflammation, such as toxins and food allergens, and removing those.

Which Lyme Brain therapies were you able to do at home on your own, and which required the help of a doctor?

I could work on diet by myself, and also prayer and exercise. I also regularly did sauna therapy and used a rebounder to keep my lymphatic system moving. I think the lymphatic system gets overlooked in treatment, but it's the system that shuttles toxins from your cells to the central veins to be excreted. It takes the trash out, so to speak. Rebounding helped, as well as body brushing.

I was on antibiotics for 1½ years, but they only made me feel worse. I didn't feel that they helped me to heal from Lyme Brain at all. They messed up my circadian rhythm, and for years, I couldn't go to sleep before 2 a.m. My friend Lee Cowden, M.D. once told me that the gut plays a big role in circadian rhythm, so I assume that was the connection.

Do you have any words of advice to Lyme patients with regards to Lyme Brain?

You have to find the cause of Lyme Brain. Diet is the easiest place to start. Remove all allergenic and inflammatory foods. Try to get exercise if you can. Expose yourself to sunlight, as it helps the brain to produce serotonin. I would suggest getting hormone and neurotransmitter testing done. And detox on a regular basis.

I also think spiritual life is so important. God can help us to get through everything that is going on in our lives and give us wisdom for all things. I recommend getting quiet and asking God to speak to you and show you what you need to do to get better, and then speak healing words over yourself.

Connie Strasheim is the author, co-author or ghostwriter of 10 wellness books, including New Paradigms in Lyme Disease Treatment: 10 Top Doctors Share Treatments that Work *(Fall, 2016) and* Insights into Lyme Disease Treatment. *She is also a medical copywriter and Editor of Pro Health's Lyme disease page as well as Editor of the Alternative Cancer Research Institute. In addition, she is a healing prayer minister. Her passion is to help people with complex chronic illnesses find freedom from disease and soul-spirit sickness using whole body medicine and prayer, and she collaborates with some of the world's best integrative doctors to do this. In addition to Lyme disease, Connie's books focus on cancer, nutrition, detoxification and spiritual healing. You can learn more about her work at: www. ConnieStrasheim.org (.com pending).*

CHAPTER 43

SANDY BERENBAUM, L.C.S.W.

Could you tell us a bit about the context in which you work with Lyme patients?

I am a licensed clinical social worker.

To give you a bit of history, many years ago I had a bad case of Lyme myself—all brain stuff, no joint pain. I was treated for four years and everything cleared, but then, four years after that, I had arthroscopic surgery on my shoulder and my symptoms returned. I don't think I would have become symptomatic again had I been put on antibiotics before and after the surgery. Dr. Horowitz is my family doctor, and when I told him of the return of symptoms, he prescribed a few more months of antibiotics. I did fine until about 2002 when toxic mold came into my life. My impression is that there are so many mold issues out there, and very few doctors really know it well. That was a whole other thing for me, and I worked with a naturopath to deal with that.

Anyway, back in 1990, I had found my way to Dr. Joseph Burrascano after six years of misdiagnosis by major physicians, including neurologists in New York City. I also started going to conferences as I realized that many doctors locally didn't know what was wrong with me. I went to two or three conferences in one year. That was 1991. Then a teenager came to see me who was psychotic. He was referred to me because his parents knew that I worked with acting-out adolescents. He was paranoid, wouldn't go to school and was psychotic. I thought he'd have to go into a psychiatric hospital if these symptoms did not improve.

At that time, I insisted that at least one parent be involved with the therapy, and be seen by my co-therapist and me. I felt tentative about suspecting that there may be a medical cause of his psychiatric symptoms because that idea was new to me, but he was so unstable that he had to be admitted to a psychiatric hospital… or could it be Lyme disease? I had just gone to a Lyme conference, and I had just learned that Lyme could affect the brain.

I suggested that his mother take him to the pediatrician, and they test him for Lyme. When the test came back negative, and the pediatrician told them it could not be Lyme, I was still troubled by the diagnosis of mental illness. I just didn't want him to go down a life-long road of medications for a psychiatric illness he might not have. I therefore suggested that his mother take him to another doctor who was more experienced with Lyme, and she agreed. I referred them to a pediatrician who began the process of treatment–a process that took years–but this young man never needed to go into a hospital. The antibiotics the doctor used crossed the blood-brain barrier, therefore tackling the infection in the brain. He is a high-functioning adult today, with a career and a young family.

Within a couple of years of treating him, the doctor was pressured into stopping this comprehensive treatment of Lyme disease that had worked so well for my young client. The medical group to which he belonged, and the hospital he was affiliated with, would end his affiliations if the doctor continued on that path. At that point, I was just beginning to see how doctors were targeted for treating Lyme disease comprehensively, rather than very short term, with reliance on a simple blood test that produced a large percentage of false negatives.

By the way, as the symptoms in his brain cleared, physical symptoms emerged. He started getting pain and other symptoms that he hadn't had before. Ultimately, it was very clear that it was Lyme disease. He went from failing everything in high school and staying home for a year and a half during high school, to college and a full scholarship to law school.

That got me thinking of other kids with issues such as anorexia nervosa and drug addiction. Every time I thought it was Lyme, I was right, and I was angered by what I was seeing. I took no pleasure in being correct, when so many doctors were wrong in their failing to appropriately diagnose and treat Lyme.

What percentage of your practice has Lyme and what percentage are kids versus adults?

100% of my clients are Lyme disease patients or family members of Lyme patients, and it's been that way for 11 years. I would say about 2/3 are kids or relatives of kids (such as mothers of kids with Lyme), and about 1/3 are adults. I often suggest that clients have a trusted note-taker in my office or on a phone session with me, such as a close friend or family member—someone who doesn't have Lyme encephalopathy ("Lyme Brain!"). Short-term memory is a major problem for patients with Lyme disease.

Do you have any specific assessment tools that you use?

Over the years, I have developed the Berenbaum Screening Protocol [see Appendix A]. I wanted a very quick and easy assessment tool to give a quick screening rather than a full assessment. This tool can help psychotherapists know when to refer for a Lyme evaluation.

I never use the phrase "Lyme testing;" it's more an evaluation, since, as ILADS puts it, Lyme disease is a "clinical diagnosis" and not one based on serology. It's not my concern how many positive bands a patient has on a Western blot. My job is to see where the patient is at and help guide them through their illness, using a problem-solving approach.

Also, in this regard, one of the issues that medical and mental health practitioners need to keep in mind is that they need to be open and keep learning. That's key. Even if you've had Lyme and your kids were sick with it and you've educated yourself about it. If you stop there, that's not enough. I believe you need to be going to Lyme conferences regularly if you practice in Lyme-endemic areas. Things change—for example, we didn't know at the beginning about co-infections, then PANDAS [Pediatric Autoimmune Neuropsychiatric Disorders Associated with Streptococcal Infections] and that connection, then the toxic mold issue. Who knows what's next?

I'm getting more and more interested in how gut issues relate to the brain, especially in terms of irritability and mood issues.

How do you work with Lyme patients? What approaches do you take?

I strongly believe that it has to be a problem-solving approach. I call what I do responsive psychotherapy. I respond to the needs that are presented to me, and work with them in my office or by phone. I have clients all over the country. I began to do telephone counseling because it was hard for Lyme patients to find a therapist who understands Lyme, and works the way I do.

One thing that comes up with kids a lot is how the schools are dealing with their illness, whether these students are provided with the appropriate accommodations, modifications and specialized instruction, due to the deficits that affect their learning. Sometimes the problem is that the parents aren't on the same page; sometimes the grandparents can interfere and cause tension. Often it is a boundary issue—parents need to establish boundaries with family members, friends and schools.

Also related to problem solving—I talk about going from victim to survivor to thriver. Often clients come to me experiencing themselves as victims. They keep going back to how misunderstood they were, and I know what that's like because I went through it for six years myself. My belief is that if I can help them get out of the victim stance, then they can start problem solving. If they stay focused on how horrible it was to be misdiagnosed by their doctors, then they can't go forward and ask, "Where are we right now?" Maybe they'll take action later, such as writing a letter to those doctors who misdiagnosed them or their children, but this is not the time. For now, they have to focus on navigating through their illness and getting well. It can't go both ways—you can't be a problem solver and a victim at the same time. You have to choose one or the other.

What I try to do is move them towards becoming problem solvers. I have to individualize it to the family and adapt depending on where the individual is and what the issue is—their marriage, their workplace, their finances, are they ever going to be able to have children?

For example, I had a patient with active Lyme who got pregnant but had an early miscarriage. But they adapted themselves and their lives to their situation, and began considering adopting older kids. There are different ways to look at life.

I also try to guide patients towards not thinking too far ahead, just taking them to where they think their next step may be. If you look too far ahead, you're not going to be able to make the decisions you need to make today, tomorrow and next month.

Do you see different co-infections manifesting with different Lyme Brain symptoms?

I had noticed a number of years ago that every kid that came in with rages had a diagnosis of Bartonella from their Lyme doctor. So I called Dr. Charles Ray Jones and asked him if there was a link between Bartonella and rages. He told me that there is, indeed, a correlation between Bartonella and rages.

Then three years ago, I went to a PANDAS conference, and that's when I started learning more about that. I'd been seeing kids with Lyme and PANDAS, and they were a piece of work! In fact, I was at Dr. Horowitz's office one time and I'd heard a child screaming. When I saw the mother in the waiting room, she was very embarrassed, as her son raced around the waiting room, not listening to her. I turned to her and said, "Lyme and PANDAS?" She looked so relieved and told me that that was his diagnosis. I told her that I'd been to conferences on PANDAS and told her not to be embarrassed about it. It was not her fault. She was relieved to be understood by someone.

Do you see Lyme Brain symptoms as temporary for most, or do you see them becoming permanent?

I'd like to say it's always temporary, and I used to say yes it is, but now we have seen more cases of it coming back or people having some ongoing issues. I tell people, "Look. What happens if you have diabetes that was diagnosed when you were 35? The questions come up—"Am I ever going to get better? Is this ever going to end?" Then you go on this great diet, and your diabetes symptoms improve. It's not that you don't have diabetes any more, but it's well managed. But then you become symptomatic again. It turns out the diet wasn't enough. It's a question of process more than product. There are a lot of illnesses that fall into that category. The bigger issue for me is, "how do I live with what I have now?" and "what does this mean for my life moving forward?" We have what we have; we're not given perfect health all the time. I just feel like that's a realistic view.

How do you think people can best help themselves?

I think people need a guide, such as someone who does therapy like me. In fact, I'm hoping that more mental health practitioners realize that if they are working in Lyme-endemic areas, they need to become more aware of the unique issues involved. One of the goals of the book I co-authored *When Your Child Has Lyme Disease: A Parent's Survival Guide*, other than being for patients themselves, is to be a resource for other therapists. There are more conferences and seminars around the country than ever before. I believe that it is important for therapists to educate themselves about the disease, or actually array of diseases, even though most of us did not expect that our profession would require us to study such a complex illness.

I also think that a Lyme-literate medical team is so important. You can go to an integrative doctor or a Western medicine doctor who knows the antibiotics well, and then go to a well-trained naturopathic doctor, too. Each of them is trained well and has their specialties, and as long as each appreciates what the other can do, you've got yourself a good medical team.

I'm also big on environmental changes, or adapting one's environment. For example, I had one person who left a kettle boiling on the stove and forgot it was there. She ended up getting a device that would boil water then automatically shut off. It might be something like a walker, any tool that helps people to live their lives and adapt to what they're experiencing. It might only be temporary, but it can make a huge difference. If you feel bad about not being able to boil a pot of water, at least with a new automatic kettle, you can make a cup of tea! They're just doing things another way. They need to pat themselves on the back for the things they can accomplish rather than feeling bad about the things they can't.

Hope is the cornerstone.

Sandy Berenbaum, L.C.S.W., B.C.D.

Sandy is a Licensed Clinical Social Worker, with a psychotherapy and family therapy practice in Middletown, CT. Her professional experience, working with Lyme disease patients and their families in her practice, goes back 25 years.

With a deep understanding of the effect of Lyme disease on children and adolescents, she often includes education advocacy in the work she does with families. Sandy has written and spoken widely on Lyme disease and has been a co-organizer of several Lyme disease conferences, including the annual seminar for mental health practitioners sponsored by Lyme Connection in Ridgefield, CT. She is a member of ILADS (International Lyme and Associated Diseases Society), and has given several presentations at ILADS annual conferences.

Sandy serves as the Children's and Mental Health Editor of the Lyme Times, a publication of lymedisease.org, and has served as consultant on various Time for Lyme and Lyme Disease Association projects. She is an advisor to Lyme Connection, and works on programming with the two co-chairs, Jennifer Reid and Karen Gaudian.

Sandy co-authored a book with Dorothy Kupcha Leland entitled "When Your Child Has Lyme Disease: A Parent's Survival Guide."

More information can be found on her website: www.lymefamilies.com and www.lymeliteratepress.com.

CHAPTER 44

ROBERT BRANSFIELD, M.D., D.L.F.A.P.A.

In your opinion, what are the key mechanisms of Lyme Brain?

I think the inflammation is mostly what affects brain function in Lyme disease.

Let me just make the point, though, that the name "Lyme" is recognizable, but it is also too restrictive. Tick-borne disease is a more accurate name, and that's what I'm talking about. Lyme disease puts it into the IDSA criteria, whereas tick-borne illness is more encompassing. Even then, tick-borne isn't necessarily accurate either, as there are opportunistic infections that are not even tick-borne. These infections become part of our microbiome whether we like it or not.

Anyway, there are a few pathways. There are multiple infections, and there are multiple contributors to the disease process besides infectious agents. There are contributors to illness and deterrents to illness (the deterrents include the treatments).

So how it affects the brain...you don't actually have pathogens themselves in the brain to have brain-related symptoms. A lot of people think that there are always pathogens in the brain tissue, and there can be, but it's not necessarily so.

Inflammatory substances can cross the blood-brain barrier and lead to gliosis, so inflammation in the brain can be the result of infection outside of the brain. In other words, infection in the periphery can cause inflammation, which can go to the brain and cause symptoms.

It depends on what part of the brain is affected, too. The cortex is more involved in cognitive function, the limbic system is more involved with emotional states and the brain stem will lead to more of the vegetative symptoms.

People compare Lyme disease with Alzheimer's disease, but it's a different type of encephalopathy. Lyme disease produces more white matter encephalopathy, whereas Alzheimer's produces a greater predominance of grey matter symptoms, so they're qualitatively different. With white matter encephalopathy, we see slower processing speeds, word-finding problems, dyslexia and so on. But the innate intelligence is intact; there's mostly slower processing. In Alzheimer's, with the grey matter issues, there is more of a permanent loss of memory. It's just a different quality to the encephalopathy. Most of the cognitive issues I see in Lyme correlate closely with levels of fatigue.

Back to inflammation…

The other thing about inflammation is that it is a good thing in early infection. The immune system is reacting to signs of danger—infections, allergies, injury. In the short term, the immune response and inflammatory response protect us and are a healthy response to danger. In chronic infection, the danger is ongoing, so the body goes into a chronic inflammatory state.

The problem is that we often don't get adaptive immunity in Lyme disease, so it goes on to chronic persistent inflammation. You also can have autoimmune processes. So the failure of adaptive immunity leads to chronic inflammation and possible autoimmunity.

Chronic inflammation is an indicator that there is still a danger to the system, still a hazard. So there is some risk to suppressing the inflammation—such as with steroids—while there is still a hazard. In this case, the infection could progress further.

Different infections also have different fingerprints within the inflammatory response—a different fingerprint of cytokines and chemokines. These chemical responses to these infections are what give rise to symptoms of depression, anhedonia, fatigue and malaise.

How do you assess Lyme Brain?

I always do an assessment based on a detailed questionnaire and a physical exam.

I put more weight on the physical exam, both physical and mental, and less testing for microbes because they are inherently immune evasive and have immune-suppressive strategies.

I have a very detailed questionnaire where I ask about every aspect of brain function—cognitive, emotional states and so on (see Appendix B).

It's hard with these kinds of symptoms, as they're viewed by some as being subjective. It's a weakness in medicine that if symptoms are categorized as subjective and non-specific they tend to be ignored, and there is a tendency to pay more attention to symptoms like joint pain. General medicine tends to ignore mental symptoms until they're very severe.

These symptoms also involve many disciplines in medicine. Rheumatologists and infectious disease docs typically aren't good at mental status exams. It's also not their area of focus; they're not looking for those symptoms.

There are several different studies that all look at the prevalence of mental symptoms—all showed similar numbers—around 90% of patients reporting cognitive issues, and around 37% reporting depressive symptoms. 90% of patients had cognitive deficits. That's a high percentage.

What medications do you find helpful for Lyme Brain?

I use a lot of memantine, which has some similarities to amantadine, an antiviral drug. It was first used in Europe as a dementia drug. When it was used to treat AIDS, it wasn't a great antiviral drug, but they found it helped with AIDS encephalopathy, especially white matter issues. It helps with processing speed, word-finding problems etc. It's also neuroprotective and reduces glutamate hyperactivity.

I use trazadone to help promote deep sleep. I use a lot of pregabalin and doxepin also. Sodium oxybate and quintiapine are more powerful medications. Sodium oxybate I find to be the most effective, but it's more powerful and has more risks and side effects.

Modafinil and armodafinil can help executive functioning. Usually executive function impairment is the first thing to be affected, but I do try to improve sleep before trying cognitive-enhancing medications. ADD meds sometimes also help focus.

I find that quite a few Lyme patients have sleep apnea. It looks like Lyme may cause that. C-PAP machines or dental appliances, and adjusting head position with sleep, should be looked at. That helps cognitive impairment by improving sleep quality.

Nuedexta is another medication that I use sometimes. It's somewhat similar to Namenda working on glutamate, but it helps more of the emotional symptoms. It was originally approved for pseudobulbar affect, and it's used for emotional lability and emotional incontinence, but this is a rarer symptom.

I use all psych meds depending on what the patient's dominant symptoms are.

In your view, what are the most important diet and lifestyle factors for helping brain function?

I think there are two key things. One is adequate sleep. There is a vicious cycle of chronic inflammation and non-restorative sleep, but one needs to sleep more when recovering from chronic illness.

The second is avoiding unremitting chronic stress. This is also hard when chronically ill. But if we can avoid chronic stress or help the body to be able to deal with chronic stress, the immune system will do a better job, and that will make treatment more effective.

From a diet standpoint, I see a lot of gluten sensitivity, lactose sensitivity and red meat allergies. Red meat allergies are mostly caused by an allergy to the lone star tick. If patients are eating foods they're intolerant to, that will increase their symptoms, including mental symptoms.

Lyme patients need to be careful of yeast overgrowth, as Lyme grows within yeast cells. High sugar diets and antibiotics can both contribute to yeast overgrowth. They also need to avoid alcohol. Most Lyme patients are alcohol intolerant, so they do stop it, but some use it to self-medicate, which sets up a vicious cycle. I do see a certain amount of substance abuse in Lyme patients involving sugar, alcohol and pain medications.

How do you feel patients can help themselves the best?

People have to reduce the stress in their lives. You can't win a battle on two fronts at once. They have to cut back on things, but I find that when they feel better, they quickly jump into things and then relapse.

I see marathon runner-type people—many of those people never recover because of stoicism. They don't pay enough attention to body signals. They push, push, push, drive, drive, drive. That is hard on the body. They need to back off and let their body heal, listen to their body signals and recover, not drive themselves into the ground.

Lyme patients often have stress intolerance. They have sensory hyperacuity and don't filter sensory input well. One study showed that this was due to an overactive thalamus, but it stresses people out because they become flooded with sensory input.

Many people experience anxiety as a new symptom with their Lyme disease, and they have a diminished tolerance for stress. Their level of functioning is less than it used to be, so they need to be aware of that and live their life accordingly—be less hyper in how they go about things. It's not easy for everyone to curtail his or her lifestyle. Many people resist that, even though it's what they need to do. Then as they get better, they need to condition themselves gradually, not plunging back in as soon as they have a good day and trigger a relapse.

How do you see Lyme Brain manifest in children?

Often children have been sick for so long they lose the sense of their baseline, of what normal is. Sometimes they don't know how sick they are or realize how impaired they are. They don't always complain about things that others complain about, including cognitive impairments.

The fluctuating nature of Lyme disease is especially hard on children. They may be able to rally in short bursts, but there is no sustainability over time. They rally, and then they burn out.

Because of their slow processing, it can take four hours to do one or two hours of homework. They run out of time to get projects done, so they cut into their sleep time, but then they get sleep deprived and their cycle gets all out of balance. Children need to adjust their schedule to make allowances for their cognitive deficits.

Can you make a few comments about PTSD and Lyme disease?

Intrusive symptoms are pivotal in PTSD—this leads to avoidance, hyperarousal and emotional numbing. Some Lyme patients get intrusive symptoms. When we look at the physiology of PTSD, we see over activity in the hippocampus and amygdala. This correlates with where we see impacts of inflammation, so chronic inflammation can provoke PTSD in susceptible individuals.

We see what appears to be PTSD without any provoking trauma. For those who do have prior trauma, Lyme can worsen the PTSD they have around that. I have also seen people develop PTSD from the Lyme itself; their experience of illness is the trauma.

There are some medications that can help with intrusive symptoms—topiramate and prazosin. Occasionally I'll use cyproheptadine for nightmares. These medications are in different classes and don't have much in common, but sometimes they'll work well.

This is an area that I want to do more research on. I'm interested in why it happens to some people and not to others.

Dr. Robert C. Bransfield, M.D., D.L.F.A.P.A. is a graduate of Rutgers College and the George Washington University School of Medicine. He completed his psychi-

atric residency training at Sheppard and Enoch Pratt Hospital. He is board certified by the American Board of Psychiatry and Neurology in Psychiatry. Dr. Bransfield's primary activity is an office-based private practice of psychiatry with an emphasis upon treatment-resistant cases.

He has held teaching appointments at Hahnemann Medical College and Eastern Virginia Medical School. He has taught in many settings to physicians, mental health professionals and the public. He has performed research and has a particular interest in psychopharmacology, a unified theory of mental health and illness, the link between microbes and mental illness, Lyme and other tick-borne disease, violence, and the link between microbes and violence.

Dr. Bransfield has authored and co-authored a number of publications in peer-reviewed literature, other medical publications and books. He has held a number of administrative positions for various organizations involved with a number of health, mental health and community related activities.

Dr. Bransfield has been active in political advocacy on a national, state and local level. He has appeared on network and regional television, radio and various publications. He has a particular interest in preserving a health care system with traditional ethics, access, privacy, freedom, quality and cost-effectiveness at a time when these critical attributes of the health care system are being threatened.

http://www.mentalhealthandillness.com/ has several articles by Dr. Bransfield. His article "Lyme Disease, Comorbid Tick-Borne Diseases, and Neuropsychiatric Disorders" was published in Psychiatric Times, vol. 24 no. 14, December 1, 2007. http://www.psychiatrictimes.com/display/article/10168/55056

CHAPTER 45

LEO SHEA, PH.D.

———∞———

Please explain to us a little about the role you play in the care of patients with Lyme disease.

My role is to evaluate the neuropsychological components of the individual through a comprehensive evaluation focusing on cognition, emotion and behavior—or in other words, how one thinks, feels and acts—and how those elements interact in the daily life of the person.

Lyme patients present with a variety of symptoms. Some present with more cognitive symptoms, others more emotional and some with behavioral aspects that impact their life. Most often, it's a mixture of all three. How one deals with the cognitive changes may generate certain emotional or behavioral characteristics that impact the way they deal with tasks and with people. For example, one may present with a sense of irritability and rage, and be highly critical, or conversely, shut down and withdraw. Others can be angered by too much stimulus in their environment, such as noise or light. Often people develop protective behaviors to avoid stimulus overload such as sitting with headphones or removing themselves from highly public environments where noise and light adversely affect them. From a cognitive standpoint, one has to evaluate such things as attention, concentration, memory, reasoning and multitasking and how they impact their ability to deal with the challenges of daily life. When I sit down with a person, I go through the list of their complaints and symptoms and talk about how such have impacted their life, and help them understand and improve their awareness of the nature of their symptoms.

Following evaluation, I meet with the patient to go over results and to structure a rehabilitative treatment regimen that will address their needs. For some, focus may be on emotions, others cognition, still others behaviors. They may need to clear some of the feelings about their experience before doing the cognitive work. Or for others, if they are manifesting certain behaviors or acting out, they will marginalize themselves further from their social environment, so that the behavior may take primary focus in the rehabilitative process.

Which have you found to be the most prominent when it comes to Lyme patients?

I have found that cognition is the most prominent weakness displayed in individuals diagnosed with Lyme. It is helpful to remind patients that a decline in cognition is a normal part of the disease, even though it feels abnormal.

The key is to help them accept their present status but gain insight into the techniques that will help them improve and return to competent functioning. We try to give people something that they feel they can achieve so that they feel they can confront the disease and move forward through the disease. Otherwise, the disease becomes central, not the person.

I also remind people that the disease is just one component of who they are, that the whole person is so much more than that. We need to understand their history. Such things as: Have they had the disease for a long time? Have they lost hope? What have they seen other people experience with the same disease? What support systems do they have that can sustain them through the process?

In your opinion, what are the key mechanisms of Lyme Brain?

We know that the infection itself does invade the sensory system and the organic system, and one needs to focus on the totality of the person rather than discrete components. We need also to help the person understand that the organic process of infection is what is producing the changes in the person's ability to function.

We also know that this disease is pervasive and can impact every system and organ in the body, and has a tropism for the GI system and the brain.

How do you see different co-infections manifesting different symptoms?

There are multiple components to each of the tick-borne diseases, and one can see greater cognition challenges in one of the diseases as compared with greater emotional/behavioral challenges in another. So, Lyme often is different from Babesia and Bartonella in the various functional components.

What do you view as the most helpful assessment tools?

Medical records, individual self-report, SPECT scans and neuropsychological testing.

The information that we're learning from sleep researchers is so important. I think that every Lyme patient should have a sleep study done by trained sleep researchers. For example, there is research done in Tampa and other military facilities with brain-injured individuals. They are giving them medications to help them sleep, but they're also finding that those same medications may exacerbate sleep problems in the long-term.

Do you find the majority of Lyme Brain symptoms to be temporary? And what proportion of patients do you feel have permanent damage?

I do think the majority of people can have significant change and return to good function, even if it's not complete restoration. I have found approximately 10-15% of those with chronic Lyme disease have continuing challenges.

I do have hope that with more awareness, addressing Lyme disease earlier than before and giving more antibiotics in the early phases of Lyme, we can prevent some of these problems from developing. I also believe that incorporating nutraceuticals and integrative medicine modalities can provide a positive impact and reduce the need for antibiotics.

How do you feel patients can help themselves the best?

I think it's crucial for people to become aware of what this illness means to them—it is a much more complex process than people understand. They receive a diagnosis, but they're not told how that diagnosis will impact all the elements of their life—job, children, marriage, sexual life, church/spiritual life and academic life. They may ask, "What is God doing to me?" and adopt a rejectionist attitude. It is important to get a holistic view of how it impacts their family, who will support them, how they can get caretakers to understand what they're going through, and how they can get family members to understand.

From a patient standpoint, it would be beneficial if the doctor gave the diagnosis and then recommended specific treatment modalities to improve their health, apart from just medication. There needs to be a comprehensive program early on, and that would increase their awareness and prove very helpful. Such a program allows the patient to have some control over their experience, rather than the illness controlling the patient.

There is also a lot of anxiety produced when patients see multiple doctors in seeking out diagnosis and treatment, and often each doctor tells them something different. This can happen in the world of Lyme disease where controversy and fractionated medical opinions can leave the patient in a quandary. It's hard for patients to know where to place their trust and belief, and in whom, and that can be very anxiety provoking.

How do you see Lyme Brain manifest in children?

If children get diagnosed quickly and get the right medication, they usually do well. The challenge is when a child is not properly diagnosed and has to go to multiple physicians. Children may start to dislike the medical profession, which makes compliance challenging, and it becomes very stressful for the family unit. As time goes on, the family's finances will be strained. Often people who do not understand Lyme disease may question whether the child is really sick or is trying to get out of school.

Psychoemotional education in children is absolutely crucial—the family must get together to be able to understand what the disease does and how it will affect the family as a unit. Then they can rally around the child and be supportive. In having such an educational process, parents and siblings will better understand the sequelae of the tick-borne illness. This education and support needs to be re-inforced from time to time, preferably every couple of months, to keep everyone sufficiently informed.

Leo J. Shea III, Ph.D. is President of Neuropsychological Evaluation and Treat-ment Services, P.C. with offices in New York City and Quincy, Massachusetts. His practice focuses on traumatic brain injury, tick-borne diseases, chronic illness, forensic work and trauma, and provides cognitive remediation and psychotherapy to individuals and families. Dr. Shea is a Senior Staff Psychol-ogist and Clinical Associate Professor of Rehabilitation Medicine at Rusk In-stitute, a division of the New York University-Langone Medical Center. Prior to his present work with tick-borne and immunological disorders, he was Assistant Director of the NYU Brain Injury Day Treatment Program. Apart from his academic and clinical responsibilities at NYU-Langone Medical Center, Dr. Shea has served as an organizational consultant to national and internation-al corporations on human resources, administrative and executive training and development, trauma response and health care issues. His clients have included both political and public institutions, such as the United Nations Development Program.

Dr. Shea is presently the President of the International Lyme and Associated Diseas-es Educational Foundation (ILADEF) and is Immediate Past President of the Interna-tional Lyme and Associated Diseases Educational Society (ILADS).

Dr. Shea holds an Ed.M. in Counseling Psychology from the Harvard Graduate School of Education, an M.A. in Hispanic Pastoral Ministry from Barry University, an M.S. in Clinical Psychology and a Ph.D. with a dual specialty in Clinical Psychology and Clinical Neuropsychology from the Miami Institute of Psychology. Apart from his academic degrees, he is a graduate of the Organizational Development and

Consultation Program at the William Alanson White Institute for Psychoanalysis, Psychiatry and Psychology.

CONCLUSION

Without a doubt, Lyme Brain is one of the hardest aspects of Lyme disease for people to overcome. I have found that it has a profound impact on peoples' sense of value and worth, and is possibly the most challenging symptom to live with.

As simply as I (and we) say "Lyme Brain," there are clearly so many more complex elements at work here. For some, the brain fog, difficulty concentrating, lack of focus and memory loss are the primary aspects. For others, there is major depression and anxiety associated with Lyme Brain, and yet for others, there are symptoms such as panic attacks and obsessive-compulsive disorder.

These symptoms can have major impacts. They can make the difference between being able to drive or not, holding down a job or not, studying or not, having kids or not, or staying in school or not. It's easier to pretend that you don't have pain or debilitating fatigue, but it's harder to pretend that your brain is functioning well.

I hope that this book has given you some guidance on what drives Lyme Brain, and more importantly, what you can do about it. Clearly, there are many different options, which can also be numerous, confusing and hard to navigate. That is why I listed some of my favorite products and formulas to help you narrow down what to do and what to take.

As always, I emphasize the role of nutrition and home-based therapies. They are not only effective, but empowering because you can put those things into place yourself without the need for a doctor. They are often the lower-cost options, too.

My prayer for you is that you find your way out of this nightmare. I pray that you find the doctors, helpers and resources to ease the pain and figure out the root causes of the complexity to help you navigate out of this situation. I pray that the governments and health agencies bring more funding, resources and acceptance to the Lyme world, and that breakthroughs happen in the treatment of Lyme disease. As a practitioner, it's equally frustrating for me to try to figure it all out as we go. I love our ILADS community and the contributions of the practitioners there, but as a doctor living in the Lyme world every day, I see an urgent need for more research to help guide our treatment protocols and give people more information on how to help themselves.

May you find ongoing healing and recovery, may you "get your brain back," and may you get this horrible Lyme thing out of your life once and for all. And finally, may you end up with greater self-knowledge and self-awareness, and be an overall healthier and wiser individual for having made the journey.

APPENDICES

Appendix A: Berenbaum Lyme Disease Screening Protocol

1. History of changes in:

    a. Behavior at home, school, the workplace or other settings

    b. School performance or attendance

    c. Sleeping and eating patterns

    d. Socialization patterns, or dramatic changes in peer group

    e. Mood

        i. Depression

        ii. Anxiety

        iii. Suicidal tendencies or gestures

        iv. New onset of intensification of PMS

2. History of changes in activity level that could be suggestive of Lyme disease.

    • Sudden loss of interest or inability to participate in activities, such as organized sports, music, dance, drama, youth group. In adults, loss of interest in social activities and hobbies.

3. A discrete point in time at which problems began.

4. History of onset of other psychiatric symptoms (panic attacks, OCD, hallucinations, cognitive and executive functioning problems) not present in early childhood, or prior to the onset of an array of symptoms.

5. History of use of psychiatric medications, with either no success in symptom reduction or a paradoxical response.

6. History of any physical illness (flu, mononucleosis, bronchitis, strep) occurring prior to start of psychiatric, learning or behavioral problems.

7. History of short-term antibiotic treatment for medical problem (strep infections, etc.) with temporary improvement in symptoms.

Appendix B: Bransfield Assessment Table

*Source: http://www.mentalhealthandillness.com/neuropsychiatric_lyme_
assessment.htm*

> **High diagnostic significance*
> *#Uncommon symptoms*

Patient Name:
Date of Birth:
Current Age:
Date:
Date of Infection:
Date of LD Diagnosis:
Date Treatment Started:
History Exposure to Endemic Area:
History of Tick Bite:
History Erythema Migrans Rash:
With Flu-Like illness:
Recurrent Erythema Migrans Rash:
Lab Findings:
Other Diagnoses Considered:
Pre-Existing Psychiatric Illness:
Pre-Existing Physical Illness:

Cognitive Symptoms
> *Attention Span (Perception)*
> *Sustained Attention*
> *Allocation of attention*
> *Distracted by Frustration*
> *Distracted by Hyperacuity*
> > **Auditory*
> > *Visual*
> > *Tactile*
> > *Olfactory*

Memory
> **Working Memory*
> **Working Spatial Memory*
> *Recent Memory*

Remote Memory
Memory Retrieval
*Slowness of retrieval
  Words
  Numbers
  Names
  Faces
  Motor sequences
  Geographical/Spatial
*Sequential Memory
  Letter reversals
  Spelling errors
  Word substitution errors
  Number reversals

Processing

*Reading comprehension
*Auditory comprehension
Processing speed
Sound localization
Transposition of laterality
*L-R confusion
Visual imagery
*Calculation
*Fluency of speech
*Stuttering
*Slurred speech
*Fluency of written language
*Handwriting
*Spatial perceptual distortions (microscopia, etc.)
Decreased body awareness
Derealization
*Optic ataxia

Imagery

Complex imagery
*Intrusive images
  Aggressive
  Sexual
  Other
Hypnagogic Hallucinations

Vivid nightmares
Illusions
Hallucinations

Thought Processes/Exec function

Time Management
Intrusive Thoughts
Unfocused concentration
Fuzzy/fog sensation
Prioritizing multiple tasks
Concentration on multiple tasks
Racing thoughts
Obsessive thoughts
Mental apathy
Abstract reasoning

Mood Symptoms

Decreased frustration tolerance
Sudden abrupt mood swings
Hypervigilance
Paranoia

Behavioral Symptoms

Disinhibition
Exaggerated startle reflex
Explosive anger
Suicidal
Homicidal
Accident-prone
Decreased social functioning
Decreased job/school performance
Marital/family difficulties
Substance abuse
Legal difficulties
Dissociative episodes
Compensatory compulsions
Dropping objects
Crying spells

Psychiatric Syndromes

Depression

*Rapid cycling bipolar
Panic disorder
Obsessive-compulsive disorder
Social phobia
Generalized anxiety
PTSD*

Oscillating Rhythms

*Impaired sleep wakefulness cycle
Not well rested in the a.m.
Insomnia
Initial
Mid
Late
Hypersomnia
Loss of 24-hour cycle
Narcolepsy
Sleep apnea*

Eating Disorder

*Anorexia
Weight loss
Non-appetite motivated*
    *Over-eating
Weight gain w/o increased food intake
Weight gain with increased food intake*

Sexual

**Decreased libido
Menstrual irregularity
Decreased capacity for pleasure
Other*

Temperature Control

*Body temperature fluctuations
Flushing
Intolerance to heat
Intolerance to cold
Decreased body temperature
Low-grade fevers
Night sweats
Chills*

Neurological
>*Headaches*
>>**Cervical radioculopathy*
>>*Migraine*
>>*Orgasm Migraine*
>>*TMJ*
>>*Tension*
>>*Cluster*
>>*Sinus*

Cranial Nerves
I. Olfactory, loss of smell, altered taste
II. Ophthalmologic
>*Blurred vision*
>**Photophobia*
>>*Bright light*
>>*Fluorescent and flicker*
>*Floaters*
>*Flashes*
>**Conjunctivitis*
>>*Eye pain*
>>*Dry eyes*
>*Papilledema*
>*Blind spots*
>*Night blindness*
>*Peripheral shadows*
>*Other*

III, IV, VI double vision or eye drifts when tired
>*Ptosis*

V. Sensory loss

*VII. Bell's Palsy

*VIII. Tinnitus
>*Hearing loss*
>*Dizziness*
>*Vertigo*
>*Motion sickness*
>*Tullio's*

IX, X Episodic loss of speech
Choking on food, difficulty swallowing

XI. SCM and trap pain and paresis

XII. Seizures
Grand mal
*Complex partial

Other Neurological
Numbness
Tingling
Sensory loss
Burning
Static electric sensation
Crawling sensation under the skin
Stabbing sensation
Paresis
Tremor
Twitching
Muscle tightness
Muscle discomfort
Myoclonic jerks
Torticollis
#Myotonia
#EPS
Ataxia
Fainting
Herniated disks
Spasticity
Romberg
Other

Other Physical Symptoms
Joint
Pain, swelling, tightness (specify joints)
Bone thinning/fractures
*Bone pain (tibia, ribs, iliac crest, sternum, clavicle, elbow etc.)
Plantar fascitis
Chronic fatigue syndrome
Fibromyalgia

Myalgia
Chondritis (ear, nose, costochondral)
Tendonitis
Carpal Tunnel

Cardiac

Heart block
MVP
Racing pulse
Episodes of rapid and slow HR
Pericarditis
Cardiomyopathy
Murmur
Hypertension
Hypertensive crisis

Pulmonary / Upper Respiratory

Air hunger
Shortness of breath
Cough
Sore throats
Swollen glands
Asthma

Gastrointestinal (GI)

Upper GI distress
Non-ulcerative dyspepsia
Irritable bowel
#Hepatitis
#Pancreatitis
#Inflammatory bowel
#Cholecyctisis
#Gall stones

Genitourinary (GU)

Genital pain
Breast pain, tenderness
Lactation
Irritable bladder
#Atrophy of genitalia
Anesthesia of genitalia

Other

> *Striae*
> *Alcohol intolerance*
> *Hair loss*
> *Thyroid dysfunction*
> *Wilson's syndrome*
> *Adrenal insufficiency*
> *Hypoglycemia*
> *Vasculitis*
> *Ankle edema*
> *Tooth pain*
> *Nose bleeds*
> *MCS*
> *Allergies*
> *Splenomegaly*
> *Ecchymosis*
> *Chronic pain*
> *ACA*
> *Lymphocytoma*

Fluctuations of Symptoms

> **Herxheimer reaction*
> **Progression of symptoms*
> **Symptoms fluctuation throughout the day*
> *Stress increases symptoms*
> *Infectious disease increase symptoms*
> *28 day cycle or longer*
> *Perimenstrual relapse*
> *Episodic relapse*
> *Antibiotics reduce symptoms*

Babesiosis screen

> *Severe headaches*
> *Sweats*
> *Chills*
> *Severe fatigue*
> *Severe muscle ache*
> *Afternoon fever*

Ehrlichiosis screen

> *Decreased white count*
> *Decreased platelet count*

Elevated lever enzymes
Splenomegaly

Treatment

Psychiatric

Medical

Oral antibiotics
IM & IV antibiotics

Other/Status/Comments

READING AND RESOURCE LIST

Section 1

The Brain that Changes Itself: Stories of Personal Triumph from the Frontiers of Brain Science by Norman Doidge, M.D.

Section 3

The Healing Power of Herbs: The Enlightened Person's Guide to the Wonders of Medicinal Plants by Michael T. Murray, N.D.

The Mood Cure: The 4-Step Program to Take Charge of Your Emotions–Today by Julia Ross.

Section 4

The Lyme Diet: Nutritional Strategies for Healing from Lyme Disease by Nicola McFadzean, N.D.

Grain Brain: The Surprising Truth About Wheat, Carbs, and Sugar–Your Brain's Silent Killers by David Perlmutter, M.D.

Brain Maker: The Power of Gut Microbes to Heal and Protect Your Brain–For Life, by David Perlmutter, M.D.

Excitotoxins: The Taste that Kills by Russell L. Blaylock, M.D.

www.russellblaylockmd.com

Section 5

Lumosity Brain Games & Brain Training: www.lumosity.com

Sudoku Puzzles: www.sudoku.com

Switch On Your Brain: The Key to Peak Happiness, Thinking, and Health by Dr. Caroline Leaf.

Who Switched Off Your Brain: Solving the Mystery of He Said/She Said by Dr. Caroline Leaf.

Dr. Leaf's 21-Day Brain Detox Program: www.21daybraindetox.com

The Biology of Belief: Unleashing the Power of Consciousness, Matter, and Miracles by Bruce H. Lipton, Ph.D.

Audio CD: *The Wisdom of Your Cells: How Your Beliefs Control Your Biology* Bruce H. Lipton, Ph.D.

Dr. Joseph Mercola: www.mercola.com

Emotional Freedom Techniques (EFT): www.emofree.com

Energy Psychology: www.energypsych.org

Psych-K by Rob Williams, MA: www.psych-k.com

Section 6

Zengar Neuroptimal: www.zengar.com

Holosync Meditation Technology: www.centerpointe.com

LifeFlow Audio Technology: www.lifeflow.net

Insight Program: www.immramma.org

Brain Tap Technologies: www.braintaptechnologies.com

Section 7

Mold Warriors: Fighting America's Hidden Health Threat by Ritchie C. Shoemaker, M.D. and James Schaller.

www.survivingmold.com

Section 8

Bipolar Kids: Helping Your Child Find Calm in the Mood Storm by Rosalie Greenberg, M.D.

When Your Child Has Lyme Disease: A Parent's Survival Guide by Sandy Berenbaum, L.C.S.W. and Dorothy Kupcha Leland.

WORKS CITED

Aalto, A, J Sjowall, L Davidsson, P Forsberg, and O Smedby. "Brain magnetic resonance imaging does not contribute to the diagnosis of chronic neuroborreliosis." *Acta Radiol* 48, no. 7 (2007): 755-762.

Agarwal, R, and G Sze. "Neuro-lyme disease: MR imaging findings." *Radiology* 253, no. 1 (October 2009): 167-73.

Aggarwal, Bharat B, Subash C Gupta, and Bokyung Sung. "Curcumin: an orally bioavailable blocker of TNF and other pro-inflammatory biomarkers." *Br J Pharmacol* 169-8 (2013): 1672-1692.

Agosta, F, M A Rocca, B Benedetti, R Capra, C Cordioli, and M Filippi. "MR imaging assessment of brain and cervical cord damage in patients with neuroborreliosis." *AJNR Am J Neuroradiol* 27, no. 4 (2006): 892-894.

Agrawal, R, and F Gomez-Pinilla. "'Metabolic syndrome' in the brain: deficiency in omega-3 fatty acid exacerbates dysfunctions in insulin receptor signalling and cognition." *J Physiol* 590, no. Pt 10 (May 2012): 2485-99.

Alhola, P, and P Polo-Kantolo. "Sleep deprivation: Impact on cognitive performance." *Neuropsychiatr Dis Treat* 3, no. 5 (2007): 553-67.

Anonymous. "Choline." *Wikipedia: The Free Encylopedia.* 2016 йил 17th-March. https://en.wikipedia.org/wiki/Choline.

Anuradha, B, and P Varalakshmi. "Protective role of DL-alpha-lipoic acid against mercury-induced neural lipid peroxidation." *Pharmacol Res* 39, no. 1 (1999): 67-80.

Audhya, T. "Advances in measurement of platelet catecholamines at Sub-picomole level for diagnosis of depression and anxiety." *Clinical Chemistry* 151, no. 6 Supplement (2005).

"Babesiosis." *Wikipedia: The Free Encyclopedia.* 2016 йил 26-February. https://en.wikipedia.org/wiki/Babesiosis.

Baggish, Aaron L, and David R Hill. "Antiparasitic Agent Atovaquone." *Antimicrob Agents Chemother* 46, no. 5 (May 2002): 1163-1173.

Banji, Othila J F, David Banji, and Kalpana Ch. "Curcumin and hesperidin improve cognition by suppressing mitochondrial dysfunction and apoptosis induced by D-galactose in rat brain." *Food Chem Toxicol* 74 (2014): 51-9.

Bar, K J, T Jochum, F Hager, W Meissner, and H Sauer. "Painful hallucinations and somatic delusions in a patient with the possible diagnosis of neuroborreliosis." *Clin J Pain* 21, no. 4 (July-August 2005): 362-3.

Bernardino, A L, D Kaushal, and M T Philipp. "The antibiotics doxycycline and minocycline inhibit the inflammatory responses to the Lyme disease spirochete Borrelia burgdorferi." *J Infect Dis* 199, no. 9 (May 2009): 1379-88.

Bjelland, Ingvar, Grethe S Tell, Stein E Vollset, Svetlana Konstantinova, and Per M Ueland. "Choline in anxiety and depression: Tthe Hordaland Health Study." *Am J Clin Nutr* 90, no. 4 (October 2009): 1056-1060.

Bourret, T J, J A Boylan, K A Lawrence, and F C Gherardini. "Nitrosative damage to free and zinc-bound cysteine thiols underlies nitric oxide toxicity in wild-type Borrelia burgdorferi." *Mol Microbiol* 81, no. 1 (July 2011): 249-73.

Bradford, Robert W, and Henry W Allen. "Biochemistry of Lyme Disease: Borrelia Burgdorferi Spirochete/Cyst." *Townsend Letter, the Examiner of Alternative Medicine.* February/March 2006.

Braniste, V, et al. "The gut microbiota influences blood-brain barrier permeability in mice." *Sci Transl Med* 6, no. 263 (November 2014): 263ra158.

Bransfield, R C. "The psychoimmunology of lyme/tick-borne diseases and its association with neuropsychiatric symptoms." *Open Neurol J*, 2012: 88-93.

Brinar, V V, and M Habek. "Rare infections mimicking MS." *Clin Nuerol Neurosurg* 112 (2010): 625-628.

Brinton, R D, et al. "Progesterone receptors: form and function in brain." *Front Neuroendocrinol* 29, no. 2 (May 2008): 313-39.

Brown Jr, J S. "Geographic correlation of schizophrenia to ticks and tick-borne encephalitis." *Schizophr Bull* 20, no. 4 (1994): 755-75.

Brown, N, and J Panksepp. "Low-dose naltrexone for disease prevention and quality of life." *Med Hypotheses* 72, no. 3 (March 2009): 333-7.

Buhner, Stephen Harrod. *Healing Lyme: Natural Healing and Prevention of Lyme Borreliosis and Its Coinfections.* San Diego: Raven Press, 2005.

Cameron, M, and S Chrubasik. "Oral herbal therapies for treating osteoarthritis." *Cochrane Summaries*, May 2014.

Cartwright, M J, S E Martin, and S T Donta. "More Evidence of Lyme Biotoxins: A Novel Toxin (Bb Tox 1) of Borrelia burgdorferi [Lyme disease]." *James Schaller, MD, MAR 50 Books & Top Journal Articles.* http://www.babesiabook.com/articles/morelymebiotoxinevidence.html (accessed 2015).

Cassilhas, R C, et al. "Spatial memory is improved by aerobic and resistance exercise through divergent molecular mechanisms." *Neurosience* 202 (January 2012): 309-17.

Centers for Disease Control and Prevention. *Autism Spectrum Disorder (ASD) Data & Sta-*

tistics. 2000-2010. http://www.cdc.gov/ncbddd/autism/data.html.

—. *Lyme Disease Graphs*. 1995-2014. http://www.cdc.gov/lyme/stats/chartstables/incidencebyagesex.html (accessed 2015 йил 15th-September).

Chang, C Y, D S Ke, and J Y Chen. "Essential fatty acids and human brain." *Acta Neurol Taiwan* 18, no. 4 (December 2009): 231-41.

Cheeke, P R, S Piacente, and W Oleszek. "Anti-inflammatory and anti-arthritic effects of yucca schidigera: A review." *J Inflamm (Lond)* 3 (2006): 6.

Chen, Y, X Xiao, C Wang, H Jiang, Z Hong, and G Xu. "Beneficial effect of tetrandrine on refractory epilepsy via suppressing P-glycoprotein." *Int J Neurosci* 125, no. 9 (2015): 703-10.

Chiu, Chi-Iso, and De-Maw Chuang. "Neuroprotective action of lithium in disorders of the central nervous system." *Zhong Nan Da Xue Xue Bao Yi Xue Ban* 36, no. 6 (June 2011): 461-476.

Chuan-Li, L, et al. "Polysaccharides from Smilax glabrae inhibit the pro-inflammatory mediators via ERK1/2 and JNK pathways in LPS-induced RAW264.7 cells." *Carbohydr Polym* 122 (May 2015): 428-436.

Cimanga, K, T De Bruyne, L Pieters, A J Vlietinck, and C A Turger. "In vitro and in vivo antiplasmodial activity of cryptolepine and related alkaloids from Cryptolepis sanguinolenta." *J Nat Prod* 60 (1997): 688-691.

Colcombe, S J, et al. "Aerobic fitness reduces brain tissue loss in aging humans." *J Gerontol A Biol Sci Med Sci* 58, no. 2 (February 2003): 176-80.

Crane, P K, et al. "Glucose levels and risk of dementia." *N Engl J Med* 369, no. 6 (August 2013): 540-8.

Daiello, L A, A Gongvatana, S Dunsiger, R A Cohen, B R Ott, and Alzheimer's Disease Neuroimaging Initiative. "Association of fish oil supplement use with preservation of brain volume and cognitive function." *Alzheimers Dement* 11, no. 2 (February 2015): 226-35.

Dean, Olivia, Frank Giorlando, and Michael Berk. "N-Acetlycysteine in psychiatry: current therapeutic evidence and potentialmechanisms of action." *J Psychiatry Neurosci*, March 2011: 78-86.

Dezmalj-Grbelja, L, R Covic-Negovetic, and V Demarin. "Differential diagnosis and diagnostic algorithm of demyelinating diseases." *Acta Clin Croat* 48, no. 3 (2009): 345-8.

Doidge, N. *The Brain That Changes Itself: Stories of Personal Triumph from the Frontiers of Brain Science*. New York: Penguin Books, 2007.

Donta, S T, R B Noto, and J A Vento. "SPECT brain imaging in chronic Lyme disease." *Clin Nucl Med*, no. 37 (September 2012): e219-22.

Durovska, J, S Bazovska, J Pancak, M Zaborska, M Derdakova, and P Traubner. "Infection with B. burgdorferi s.l., and the CNS demyelinating disease. A case report." *Neuro Endocrinol Lett* 32, no. 4 (2011): 411-4.

Edmonds, Caroline J, Rosanna Crombie, and Mark R Gardner. "Subjective thirst moderates changes in speed of responding associated with water consumption." *Front Hum Neurosci*, July 2013.

Elsheikha, H M, and N A Khan. "Protozoa traversal of the blood-brain barrier to invade the central nervous system." *FEMS Microbiol Rev* 34, no. 4 (July 2010): 532-53.

eMed Expert. "eMed Expert Comparisions." *Doxycycline versus minocycline*. http://www.emedexpert.com/compare-meds/doxycycline-vs-minocycline.shtml (accessed 2015).

Esmon, C T. "The interactions between inflammation and coagulation." *Br J Haematol* 131, no. 4 (November 2005): 417-30.

Evans, J D, T F Jacobs, and E W Evans. "Role of acetyl-L-carnitine in the treatment of diabetic peripheral neuropathy." *Ann Pharmacother* 42, no. 11 (November 2008): 1686-91.

Fallon, B A, and J A Nields. "Lyme disease: a neuropsychiatric illness." *Am J Psychiatry* 151, no. 11 (November 1994): 1571-83.

Fallon, B A, et al. "Regional cerebral blood flow and metabolic rate in persistent Lyme encephalopathy." *Arch Gen Psychiatry* 66, no. 5 (May 2009): 554-63.

Fernandez, R E, M Rothberg, G Ferencz, and D Wujack. "Lyme Disease of the CNS: MR imaging findings in 14 cases." *AJNR Am J Neuroradiol* 11, no. 3 (1990): 479-481.

Forsgren, S. "Kryptopyrroluria (aka Hemopyrrollactamuria): A Major Piece of the Puzzle in Overcoming Chronic Lyme Disease." *Explore* 18, no. 6 (2009).

Fritzsche, M. "Seasonal correlation of sporadic schizophrenia to Ixodes ticks and Lyme borreliosis." *Int J Health Geogr* 1, no. 1 (2002): 2.

Garcia-Monco, J C, and J L Benach. "Mechanisms of injury in Lyme neuroborreliosis." *Semin Neurol* 17, no. 1 (March 1997): 57-62.

George, T I, G Manley, J E Koehler, V S Hung, M McDermott, and A Bollen. "Detection of Bartonella henselae by polymerase chain reaction in brain tissue of an immunocompromised patient with mutliple enhancing lesions. Case report and review of the literature." *J Neurosurg* 89, no. 4 (1998): 640-4.

Gerber, J E, J E Johnson, M A Scott, and K T Madhusudhan. "Fatal meningitis and encephalitis due to Bartonella henselae bacteria." *J Forensic Sci* 47, no. 3 (May 2002): 640-4.

Gomez-Pinilla, F, S Vaynman, and Z Ying. "Brain-derived neurotrophic factor functions as a metabotrophin to mediate the effects of exercise on cognition." *Eur J Neurosci* 28, no. 11 (December 2008): 2278-87.

Gould, E, A J Reeves, M S Graziano, and C G Gross. "Neurogenesis in the Neocortex of Adult Primates." *Science* 286 (October 1999).

Greenberg, H E, G Ney, S M Scharf, L Ravdin, and E Hilton. "Sleep quality in Lyme disease." *Sleep* 18, no. 10 (December 1995): 912-6.

Greenberg, Rosalie. *Bipolar Kids: Helping Your Child Find Calm in the Mood Storm.* Boston: DeCapo Press, 2008.

—. "Tick-Borne Diseases and the Brain: Implications for Pediatric Psychiatry." *ILADS Conference 2014.* Washington, DC, 2014 йил 10th-October.

Hadjivassiliou, M, D S Sanders, R A Grunewald, N Woodroofe, S Boscolo, and D Aeschlimann. "Gluten sensitivity: from gut to brain." *Lancet Neurol* 9, no. 3 (March 2010): 318-30.

Hadjivassiliou, M, et al. "Clinical, radiological, neurophysiological, and neuropathological characteristics of gluten ataxia." *Lancet* 352, no. 9140 (November 1998): 1582-5.

Henderson, V W, et al. "Cognition, mood, and physiological concentrations of sex hormones in the early and late menopause." *PNAS* 110, no. 50 (December 2013): 20290-20295.

Hucklenbroich, Joerg, et al. "Aromatic-turmerone induces neural stem cell proliferation in vitro and in vivo." *Stem Cell Res Ther* 5, no. 4 (September 2014): 100.

Jackson, Jessica R, William W Eaton, Nicola G Cascella, Alessio Fasano, and Deanna L Kelly. "Neurologic and Psychiatric Manifestations of Celiac Disease and Gluten Sensitivity." *Psychiatr Q* 83, no. 1 (March 2012): 91-102.

Jernigan, David. "Lyme-Induced Leaky Brain Syndrome." *Dr. David Jernigan, Hansa Center: Advanced Alternative Healthcare for Chronic Illness. Changing Lives, Not Just Bodies.™.* http://davidjernigan.blogspot.com/search?q=ammonia+ (accessed 2015).

—. "The Alkaline Brain: Lyme Borrelia-induced Hyper ammonemia." *Jernigan Neutraceuticals.* 2016. www.jnutra.com/Ammonia.html (accessed 2015).

Karakula-Juchnowicz, H, et al. "The role of IgG hypersensitivity in the pathogenesis and therapy of depressive disorders." *Nutr Neurosci.* 2014 30th-September.

Karimzadeh, F, et al. "Anticonvulsant and neuroprotective effects of Pimpinella anisum in rat brain." *BMC Complement Altern Med* 12, no. 76 (June 2012): 76.

Kesler, Shelli, et al. "Cognitive Training for Improving Executive Function in Chemotherapy-Treated Breast Cancer Survivors." *Clinical Breast Cancer* 13, no. 4 (August 2013): 299-306.

Kessler, R C, W T Chiu, O Demler, K R Merikangas, and E E Walters. "Prevalence, severity, and comorbidity of 12-month DSM-IV disorders in the National Comorbidity Survey Replication." *Arch Gen Psychiatry* 62, no. 6 (July 2005): 617-27.

Killgore, W D. "Effects of sleep deprivation on cognition." *Prog Brain Res* 185 (2010): 105-29.

Kimmatkar, N, V Thawani, L Hingorani, and R Khiyani. "Efficacy and tolerability of Boswellia serrata extract in treatment of osteoarthritis of knee-randomized double blind placebo controlled trial." *Phytomedicine* 10, no. 1 (January 2003): 3-7.

Kirby, G C, A Paine, D C Warhurst, B K Noamesi, and J D Phillipson. "In vitro and in vivo antimalarial activity of cryptolepine, a plant-derived indoloquinoline." *Phytother Res* 9 (1995): 359-363.

Klinkhammer, P, B Szelies, and W D Heiss. "Effect of phosphatidylserine on cerebral glucose metabolism in Alzheimer's disease. Dementia." *Dementia* 1, no. 4 (1990): 197-201.

Kodali, M, V K Parihar, B Hattiangady, B Shuai, and A K Shetty. "Resveratrol prevents age-related memory and mood dysfunction with increased hippocampal neurogenesis and microvasculature, and reduced glial activation." *Sci Rep* 5 (January 2015): 8075.

Kolotushkina, E V, M G Moldavan, K Y Voronin, and G G Skibo. "The influence of Hericium erinaceus extract on myelination process in vitro." *Fiziol Zh* 49, no. 1 (2003): 38-45.

Kruger, H, E Heim, B Schuknecht, and S Scholz. "Acute and chronic neuroborreliosis with and without CNS involvement: a clinical, MRI, and HLA study of 27 cases." *J Neurol* 238, no. 5 (1991): 271-280.

Lampit, Amit, Harry Hallock, and Michael Valenzuela. "Computerized Cognitive Training in Cognitively Healthy Older Adults: A Systematic Review and Meta-Analysis of Effect Modifiers." *PLoS Medicine*, November 2014.

Larson, E B, et al. "Exercise is associated with reduced risk for incident dementia among persons 65 years of age and older." *Ann Intern Med* 144, no. 2 (January 2006): 73-81.

Leaf, Caroline. "Controlling Your Toxic Thoughts." *Dr. Leaf.* 2016. http://drleaf.com/about/toxic-thoughts/.

Lee, Jiunn-Tay, Jan Xu, Jin-Moo Lee, and Grace Ku. "Amyloid- peptide induces oligodendrocyte death by activating the neutral sphingomyelinase–ceramide pathway." *J Cell Biol* 164, no. 1 (January 2004): 123-131.

Lehmann, M, B Regland, K Blennow, and C G Gottfries. "Vitamin B12-B6-folate treatment improves blood-brain barrier function in patients with hyperhomocysteinaemia and mild cognitive impairment." *Dement Geriatr Cogn Disord* 16, no. 3 (2003): 145-50.

Leite, L M, et al. "Anti-inflammatory properties of doxycycline and minocycline in experimental models: an in vivo and in vitro comparative study." *Inflammapharmacology* 19, no. 2 (April 2011): 99-110.

Leucht, S, W Kissling, and J McGrath. "Lithium for schizophrenia revisited: a systematic review and meta-analysis of randomized controlled trials." *J Clin Psychiatry* 65, no. 2 (Feb 2004): 177-86.

Liu, Y, R Mittal, N V Solis, N V Prasadarao, and S G Filler. "Mechanisms of Candida albicans Trafficking to the Brain." *PLoS Pathog* 7, no. 10 (2011): e1002305.

MacDonald, A B, and J B Miranda. "Concurrent neocortical borreliosis and Alzheimer's disease." *Hum Pathol* 18, no. 7 (Jul 1987): 759-761.

Maggioni, M, et al. "Effects of Phosphatidylserine Therapy in Geriatric Patients With Depressive Disorders." *Acta Psychiatr Scand* 81 (1990): 265-270.

McBride, Judy. "B12 Deficiency May Be More Widespread Than Thought." *United States Department of Agriculture Agricultural Research Service.* 2000   2nd-August. http://www.ars.usda.gov/is/pr/2000/000802.htm.

McCabe-Sellers, Beverly J, Cathleen G Staggs, and Margaret L Bogle. "Tyramine in foods and monoamine oxidase inhibitor drugs: A crossroad where medicine, nutrition, pharmacy, and food industry converge." *Journal of Food Composition and Analysis* 19 (2006): S58-S65.

McCaddon, A, et al. "Alzheimer's disease and total plasma aminothiols." *Biol Psychiatry* 53, no. 3 (February 2003): 254-60.

McNamara, Robert K, et al. "Docosahexaenoic acid supplementation increases prefrontal cortex activation during sustained attention in healthy boys: a placebo-controlled, dose-ranging, functional magnetic resonance imaging study." *Am J Clin Nutr* 91, no. 4 (April 2010): 1060-1067.

Miklossy, J. "Alzheimer's disease-a neurospirochetosis. Analysis of the evidence following Koch's and Hill's criteria." *J Neuroinflammation* 8 (Aug 2011): 90.

Miklossy, J, et al. "Beta-amyloid deposition and Alzheimer's type changes induced by Borrelia spirochetes." *Neurobiol Aging* 27 (2006): 228-236.

Miklossy, J, et al. "Borrelia burgdorferi persists in the brain in chronic lyme neuroborreliosis and may be associated with Alzheimer disease." *J Alzheimers Dis* 6, no. 6 (Dec 2004): 673-681.

Miklossy, J, S Kasas, A D Zurn, S McCall, S Yu, and P L McGeer. "Persisting atypical and cystic forms of Borrelia burgdorferi and local imflammation in Lyme neuroborreliosis." *J Neuroinflammation* 5, no. 4 (2008).

Misra, U K, J Kalita, and A Das. "Vitamin B12 deficiency neurological syndromes: a clinical MRI and electrodiagnostic study." *Electromyogr Clin Neurophysiol* 43 (2003): 57-64.

Mohagheghi, F, M R Bigdeli, B Rasoulian, P Hashemi, and M R Pour. "The neuroprotective effect of olive leaf extract is related to improved blood-brain barrier permeability and brain edema in rat with experimental focal cerebral ischemia." *Phytomedicine*, January 2011: 18(2-3):170-5.

Montagne, Axel, et al. "Blood-Brain Barrier Breakdown in the Aging Human Hippocampus." *Neuron* 85, no. 2 (January 2015): 296-302.

Montgomery, P, J R Burton, R P Sewell, T F Spreckelsen, and A J Richardson. "Low Blood Long Chain Omega-3 Fatty Acids in UK Children Are Associated with Poor Cognitive Performance and Behavior: A Cross-Sectional Analysis from the DOLAB Study." *PLoS ONE* 8, no. 6 (2013): e66697.

Mori, K, S Inatomi, K Ouchi, Y Azumi, and T Tuchida. "Improving effects of the mushroom Yamabushitake (Hericium erinaceus) on mild cognitive impairment: a double blinded, placebo controlled clinical trial." *Phytother Res* 23 (2009): 367-372.

Mori, K, Y Obara, T Moriya, S Inatomi, and N Nakahata. "Effects of Hericium erinaceus on amyloid (25-35) peptide-induced learning and memory deficits in mice." *Biomed Res* 32, no. 1 (2011): 67-72.

Murray, Michael T. *The Healing Power of Herbs: The Enlightened Person's Guide to the Wonders of Medicinal Plants*. 2nd. Rocklin: Prima Publishing, 1995.

Myers, T A, D Kaushal, and M T Phillip. "Microglia are mediators of Borrelia burgdorferi-induced apoptosis in SH-SY5Y neuronal cells." *PLos Pathog* 5, no. 11 (November 2009): e1000659.

Nagamatsu, L S, et al. "Physical activity improves verbal and spatial memory in older adults with probable mild cognitive impairment: a 6-month randomized controlled trial." *J Aging Res* 2013 (2013): 861893.

Nagano, M, et al. "Reduction of depression and anxiety by 4 weeks Hericium erinaceus intake." *Biomed Res* 31, no. 4 (2010): 231-7.

Nazario, J, and D P Kuffler. "Hyperbaric oxygen therapy and promoting neurological recovery following nerve trauma." *Undersea Hyperb Med* 38, no. 5 (September-October 2011): 345-66.

"Neurotransmitter." *Wikipedia: The Free Encyclopedia*. 2016 1st-March. http://en.wikipedia.org/wiki/Neurotransmitter.

Noguchi, H, and J W Moore. "A demonstration of Treponema Pallidum in the brain in cases of general paralysis." *J Exp Med* 17, no. 2 (1913): 232-238.

Nutramedix: Bionatus Laboratories. "Pinella: Brain/Nerve Cleanse." *Bionatus Nutramedix News and Research*. http://www.nutramedix.ec/pdfs/Pinella_flyer.pdf (accessed 2015).

O'Brien, J S, and E L Sampson. "Lipid composition of the normal human brain: gray matter, white matter, and myelin." *J Lipid Res* 6, no. 4 (October 1965): 537-44.

Oksi, J, et al. "Inflammatory brain changes in Lyme borreliosis. A report on three patients and review of literature." *Brain* 119 (Pt 6) (December 1996): 2143-54.

Packer, L, H J Tritschler, and K Wessel. "Neuroprotection by the metabolic antioxidant alpha-lipoic acid." *Free Radic Biol Med* 22, no. 1-2 (1997): 359-78.

Park, J, K S Choi, D J Grab, and J S Dumler. "Divergent interactions of Ehrlichia chaffeensis-and Anaplasma phagocytophilum-infected leukocytes with endothelial cell barriers." *Infect Immun* 71, no. 12 (December 2003): 6728-33.

Park, Y S, J H Lee, J Bondar, J A Harwalkar, H Safayhi, and M Golubic. "Cytotoxic action of acetyl-11-keto-beta-boswellic acid (AKBA) on meningioma cells." *Planta Med* 68, no. 5 (2002): 397-401.

Pascual-Leone, A, A Amedi, F Fregni, and L B Merabet. "The plastic human brain cortex." *Annu Rev Neurosci* 28 (2005): 377-401.

Paslakis, G, W F Blum, and M Deuschle. "Intranasal insulin-like growth factor I (IGF-I) as a plausible future treatment of depression." *Med Hypotheses* 79, no. 2 (August 2012): 222-5.

Petaga, J. "Inflammation and coagulation. An overview." *Thromb Res* 127 , no. Suppl 2 (January 2011): S34-7.

Picard, Richard. "Bartonella: a Stealth Infection " *Dr Richard Picard: Redefining Wellness.* 2015 29-March. http://www.nutritionalhealthnow.com/bartonella-a-stealth-infection/.

Plane, Jennifer M, Yan Shen, David E Pleasure, and Wenbin Deng. "Prospects for Minocycline Neuroprotection." *Arch Neurol* 67, no. 12 (December 2010): 1442-1448.

Pohl-Koppe, A, K E Balashov, A C Steere, E L Logigan, and D A Hafler. "Identification of a T cell subset capable of both IFN-gamma and IL-10 secretion in patients with chronic Borrelia burgdorferi infection." *J Immunol* 160, no. 4 (February 1998): 1804-10.

Pottala, J V, K Yaffe, J G Robinson, M A Espeland, R Wallace, and W S Harris. "Higher RBC EPA + DHA corresponds with larger total brain and hippocampal volumes: WHIMS-MRI study." *Neurology* 82, no. 5 (February 2014): 435-42.

Rabbitt, P, et al. "Losses in gross brain volume and cerebral blood flow account for age-related differences in speed but not in fluid intelligence." *Neuropsychology* 20, no. 5 (September 2006): 549-57.

Radak, Z, S Kumagai, A W Taylor, H Naito, and S Goto. "Effects of exercise on brain function: role of free radicals." *Appl Physiol Nutr Metab* 32, no. 5 (October 2007): 942-6.

Rai, Balwant, Jasdeep Kaur, Reinhilde Jacobs, and Jaipaul Singh. "Curcumin exhibits anti-pre-cancer activity by increasing levels of vitamin C and E, and preventing lipid peroxidation and oxidative damage." *J Oral Sci* 52, no. 2 (2010): 251-6.

Ramesh, G, L Santana-Gould, F M Inglis, J D England, and M T Philipp. "The Lyme disease spirochete Borrelia burgdorferi induces inflammation and apoptosis in cells from dorsal root ganglia." *J Neuroinflammation* 10 (July 2013): 88.

Ratajczak-Wrona, W, et al. "Nitric oxide in Lyme borreliosis. Evaluation of serum levels of nitric oxide and its biomarkers in patients with Lyme borreliosis." *Prog Health Sci* 3 (2013): 2.

Ratey, J J, and J F Loehr. "The positive impact of physical activity on cognition during adulthood: a review of underlying mechanisms, evidence and recommendations." *Rev Neurosci* 22, no. 2 (2011): 171-85.

Rissenberg, M, and S Chambers. "Distinct pattern of cognitive impairment noted in study of Lyme patients." *Lyme Times* 20 (Jan-Mar 1998): 29-32.

Riviere, G R, K H Riviere, and K S Smith. "Molecular and immunological evidence of oral Treponema in the human brain and their association with Alzheimer's disease." *Oral Microbiol Immunol* 17, no. 2 (Apr 2002): 113-8.

Roelcke, U, W Barnett, E Wilder-Smith, D Sigmund, and W Hacke. "Untreated neuroborreliosis: Bannwarth's syndrome evolving into acute schizophrenia-like psychosis. A case report." *J Neurol* 239, no. 3 (1992): 129-31.

Rolain, J M, D Arnoux, D Parzy, J Sampol, and D Raoult. "Experimental infection of human erythrocytes from alcoholic patients with Bartonella quintana." *Ann N Y Acad Sci* 990 (June 2003): 605-11.

Ross, Julia. *The Mood Cure: The 4-Step Program to Take Charge of Your Emotions--Today.* New York: Penguin Books, 2003.

Ruan, L, H S Huang, W X Jin, H M Chen, X J Li, and Q J Gong. "Tetrandrine attenuated cerebral ischemia/reperfusion injury and induced differential proteomic changes in a MCAO mice model using 2-D DIGE." *Neurochem Res* 38, no. 9 (September 2013): 1871-9.

Sapi, Eva, et al. "Evaluation of in-vitro antibiotic susceptibility of different morphological forms of Borrelia burgdorferi." *Infect Drug Resist* 4 (2011): 97-113.

Schaller, J L, G A Burkland, and P J Langhoff. "Do Bartonella Infections Cause Agitation, Panic Disorder, and Treatment-Resistant Depression?" *MedGenMed* 9, no. 3 (2007): 54.

Schrauzer, G N, and K P Shrestha. "Lithium in drinking water and the incidences of crimes, suicides, and arrests related to drug addictions." *Biol Trace Elem Res* 25, no. 2 (May 1990): 105-13.

Seiler, K P, Z Vavrin, E Eichwald, Jr., J B Hibbs, and J J Weis. "Nitric oxide production during murine Lyme disease: lack of involvement in host resistance or pathology." *Infect Immun* 63, no. 10 (October 1995): 3886-3895.

Sershen, H, Jr., L G Harsing, M Banay-Schwartz, A Hashim, M T Ramacci, and A Lajtha. "Effect of acetyl-L-carnitine on the dopaminergic system in aging brain." *J Neurosci Res* 30, no. 3 (November 1991): 555-9.

Smeland, O B, T W Meisingset, K Borges, and U Sonnewald. "Chronic acetyl-L-carnitine alters brain energy metabolism and increases noradrenaline and serotonin content in healthy mice." *Neurochem Int* 61, no. 1 (July 2012): 100-7.

Smith, Melinda, Lawrence Robinson, and Jeanne Segal. "Anxiety Medication: What You Need to Know About Anti-Anxiety Drugs." *HELPGUIDE.ORG.* 2016 йил January. http://www.helpguide.org/articles/anxiety/anxiety-medication.htm.

Soloski, M J, L A Crowder, L J Lahey, C A Wagner, W H Robinson, and J N Aucott. "Serum inflammatory mediators as markers of human Lyme disease activity." *PLos One* 9, no. 4 (April 2014): e93243.

Sood, P K, U Nahar, and B Nehru. "Curcumin attenuates aluminum-induced oxidative stress and mitochondrial duysfunction in rat brain." *Neurotox Res* 20, no. 4 (2011): 351-61.

Spencer, C M, and K L Goa. "Atovaquone. A review of its pharmacological properties and therapeutic efficacy in opportunistic infections." *Drugs* 50, no. 1 (1995): 176-96.

"Spinal Fluid and Brain Tests." *Lyme and Tick-Borne Diseaes Research Center.* http://www.columbia-lyme.org/patients/ld_spinal_fluid.html.

Sun, Q Q, S S Xu, J L Pan, H M Guo, and W Q Cao. "Huperzine-A capsules enhance memory and learning performance in 34 pairs of matched adolescent students." *Zhongguo Yao Li Xue Bao* 20, no. 7 (July 1999): 601-3.

Sweet, Richard L, and Ronald S Gibbs. *Infectious Diseases of the Female Genital Tract.* 4th. Philadelphia: Lippincott Williams & Wilkins, 2001.

Szakall, S, et al. "Cerebral effects of a single dose of intravenous vinpocetine in chronic stroke patients: a PET study." *J Neuroimaging* 8, no. 4 (October 1998): 197-204.

Szilágyi G, Nagy Z, Balkay L, Boros I, Emri M, Lehel S, Márián T, Molnár T, Szakáll S, Trón L, Bereczki D, Csiba L, Fekete I, Kerényi L, Galuska L, Varga J, Bönöczk P, Vas A, Gulyás B. "Effects of vinpocetine on the redistribution of cerebral blood flow and glucose metabolism in chronic ischemic stroke patients: a PET study." *J Neurol Sci* 229-230 (March 2005): 275-284.

Tangney, C C, et al. "Vitamin B12, cognition, and brain MRI measures: a cross-sectional examination." *Neurology* 77, no. 13 (September 2011): 1276-82.

Thadani, Vijay. "2011 Lyme and Tick Borne-Diseases National Conference." *Lyme and Tick-borne Diseases Research Center.* 2011 йил 1-2-October. http://www.columbia-lyme.org/research/scientific.html.

"Thought." *Wikipedia*. 2015 йил 18-December. https://en.wikipedia.org/wiki/Thought (accessed 2015 4th-August).

Toklu, H Z, T Hakan, N Biber, S Solakoğlu S, A V Oğünç, and G Sener. "The protective effect of alpha lipoic acid against traumatic brain injury in rats." *Free Radic Res* 43, no. 7 (2009): 658-67.

Traina, G, G Federighi, M Macchi, R Bernardi, M Durante, and M Brunelle. "Modulation of Myelin Basic Protein Gene Expression by Acetyl-l-Carnitine." *Mol Neurobiol* 44, no. 1 (August 2011): 1-6.

Varanat, M, R G Maggi, K E Linder, and E B Breitschwerdt. "Infection of human brain vascular pericytes (HBPVs) by Bartonella henselae." *Med Microbiol Immunol* 202, no. 2 (April 2013): 143-51.

Wan, Xiao-hua, Yu-wen Li, and Xiao-ping Luo. "Curcumin attenuated the lipid peroxidation and apoptotic liver injury in copper-overloaded rats." *Zhonghua Er Ke Za Zhi* 45, no. 8 (August 2007): 604-8.

Wang, R, H Yan, and X C Tang. "Progress in studies of huperzine A, a natural cholinesterase inhibitor from Chinese herbal medicine." *Acta Pharmacol Sin* 27, no. 1 (January 2006): 1-26.

Weber, C C, K Reising, W E Muller, M Schubert-Zsilavecz, and M Abdel-Tawab. "Modulation of PGP Function by Boswellic Acids." 72, no. 6 (May 2006): 507-13.

Winking, M, S Sarikaya, S Rahmanian, A Jodicke, and D K Boker. "Boswellic acids inhibit glioma growth: a new treatment option?" *J Neurooncol* 46 (2000): 97-103.

Witte, A V, L Kerti, D S Margulies, and A Floel. "Effects of resveratrol on memory performance, hippocampal functional connectivity, and glucose metabolism in healthy older adults." *J Neurosci* 34, no. 23 (June 2014): 7862-70.

Wright, D W, et al. "ProTECT: a randomized clinical trial of progesterone for acute traumatic brain injury." *Ann Emerg Med* 49, no. 4 (April 2007): 391-402, 402.e1-2.

Wu, A, E E Noble, E Tyagi, Z Ying, Y Zhuang, and F Gomez-Pinilla. "Curcumin boosts DHA in the brain: Implications for the prevention of anxiety disorders." *Biochim Biophys Acta* 1852, no. 5 (May 2015): 951-61.

Xia, D, X Yu, S Liao, Q Shao, H Mou, and W Ma. "Protective effect of Smilax glabra extract against lead-induced oxidative stress in rats." *J Ethnopharmacol* 130, no. 2 (July 2010): 414-20.

Xue, Y, Y Wang, D C Feng, B G Xiao, and L Y Xu. "Tetrandrine suppresses lipopolysaccharide-induced microglial activation by inhibiting NF-kappaB pathway." *Acta Pharmacol Sin* 29, no. 2 (February 2008): 245-51.

Yang, K, G Jin, and J Wu. "The neuropharmacology of (-)-stepholidine and its potential applications." *Curr Neuropharmacol* 5, no. 4 (December 2007): 289-94.

Zajkowska, J M, and T Hermanowska-Szpakowicz. "New aspects of the pathogenesis of lyme disease." *Przegl Epidemiol* 56, no. Suppl 1 (2002): 57-67.

Zeisel, S H, and Kerry-Ann da Costa. "Choline: An Essential Nutrient for Public Health." *Nutr Rev* 67, no. 11 (November 2009): 615-23.

ABOUT THE AUTHOR

Dr. Nicola McFadzean Ducharme is the Founder and Medical Director of RestorMedicine, an integrative medical center based in San Diego, CA. Having done her naturopathic training and completed her Bachelor of Health Sciences in Australia, she moved to the United States and obtained her Doctorate of Naturopathic Medicine from Bastyr University, starting a private practice in Southern California soon thereafter.

Dr. Nicola is a Lyme-literate Naturopathic Doctor, combining conventional and integrative approaches to treating Lyme and other tick-borne illness. She is a member of the International Lyme and Associated Diseases Society (ILADS) and has completed the ILADS Physician Training Program under the mentorship of Steven Harris, MD.

Dr. Nicola is the author of *The Lyme Diet: Nutritional Strategies for Healing From Lyme Disease, Lyme Disease in Australia: Fundamentals of an Emerging Epidemic,* and *The Beginner's Guide to Lyme Disease: Diagnosis and Treatment Made Simple.* She is also a chapter contributor to two Lyme disease books written by health care journalist Connie Strasheim, *Insights Into Lyme Disease Treatment: 13 Lyme-literate Health Care Practitioners Share Their Healing Strategies,* and *New Paradigms in Lyme Disease Treatment: 10 Top Doctors Reveal Healing Strategies That Work.*

She conducts Lyme disease clinics in Australia twice a year, helping Lyme sufferers navigate the testing and treatment options for tick-borne illness; and has been a Medical Advisor to the Lyme Disease Association of Australia.

Consultations with Dr. Nicola are scheduled through RestorMedicine's home office in San Diego. RestorMedicine can be contacted via phone at 1 (619) 546 4065 or by email – info@restormedicine.com. Patients can also schedule their own appointments online by going to www.Restormedicine.com and following the "schedule a consultation" link. Dr. Nicola works with patients both throughout the United States and internationally via telephone or Skype.

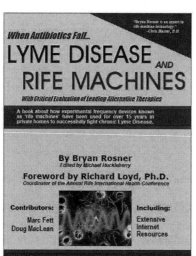

Book • $35

When Antibiotics Fail: Lyme Disease And Rife Machines, With Critical Evaluation Of Leading Alternative Therapies

By Bryan Rosner
Foreword by Richard Loyd, Ph.D.

There are enough books and websites about what Lyme disease is and which ticks carry it. But there is very little useful information for people who actually have a case of Lyme disease that is not responding to conventional antibiotic treatment. Lyme disease sufferers need to know their options, not how to identify a tick.

This book describes how experimental electromagnetic frequency devices known as rife machines have been used for over 15 years in private homes to fight Lyme disease. Also included are evaluations of more than 25 conventional and alternative Lyme disease therapies, including:

- Homeopathy
- IV and oral antibiotics
- Mercury detox.
- Hyperthermia / saunas
- Ozone and oxygen
- Samento®
- Colloidal Silver
- Bacterial die-off detox.

- Colostrum
- Magnesium supplementation
- Hyperbaric oxygen chamber (HBOC)
- ICHT Italian treatment
- Non-pharmaceutical antibiotics
- Exercise, diet and candida protocols
- Cyst-targeting antibiotics
- The Marshall Protocol®

Many Lyme disease sufferers have heard of rife machines, some have used them. But until now, there has not been a concise and organized source to explain how and why they have been used by Lyme patients. In fact, this is the first book ever published on this important topic.

The Foreword for the book is by Richard Loyd, Ph.D., coordinator of the annual Rife International Health Conference. The book takes a practical, down-to-earth approach which allows you to learn about*:

> "This book provides life-saving insights for Lyme disease patients."
>
> **- Richard Loyd, Ph.D.**

- Antibiotic treatment problems and shortcomings—why some people choose to use rife machines after other therapies fail.
- Hypothetical treatment schedules and sessions, based on the author's experience.
- The experimental machines with the longest track record: High Power Magnetic Pulser, EMEM Machine, Coil Machine, and AC Contact Machine.
- Explanation of the "herx reaction" and why it may indicate progress.
- The intriguing story that led to the use of rife machines to fight Lyme disease 20 years ago.
- Antibiotic categories and classifications, with pros and cons of each type of drug.
- Visit our website to read <u>FREE EXCERPTS</u> from the book!

Disclaimer: *Your treatment decisions must be made under the care of a licensed physician. Rife machines are not FDA approved and the FDA has not reviewed or approved of these books. The author is a layperson, not a doctor, and much of the content of these books is a statement of opinion based on the author's personal experience and research.*

Paperback book, 8.5 x 11", 203 pages, $35

The Top 10 Lyme Disease Treatments: Defeat Lyme Disease With The Best Of Conventional And Alternative Medicine

By Bryan Rosner
Foreword by James Schaller, M.D.

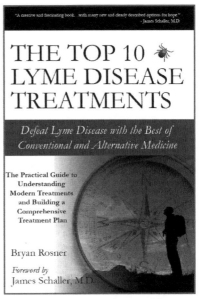

"A creative and fascinating book...with many new and clearly described options for hope."
- James Schaller, M.D.

THE TOP 10 🦟
LYME DISEASE
TREATMENTS

Defeat Lyme Disease with the Best of Conventional and Alternative Medicine

The Practical Guide to
Understanding
Modern Treatments
and Building a
Comprehensive
Treatment Plan

Bryan Rosner

Foreword by
James Schaller, M.D.

Book • $35

This information-packed book identifies ten promising conventional and alternative Lyme disease treatments and gives practical guidance on integrating them into a comprehensive treatment plan that you and your physician can customize for your individual situation and needs.

The book was not written to replace Bryan Rosner's first book (*Lyme Disease and Rife Machines*, opposing page). It was written to complement that book, offering Lyme sufferers many new foundational and supportive treatment options, based on the author's extensive research and years of personal experience. Topics include*:

- Systemic enzyme therapy, which helps detoxify tissues and blood, reduce inflammation, stimulate the immune system, and kill Lyme disease bacteria.
- Lithium orotate, a powerful yet all-natural mineral (belonging to the same mineral group as sodium and potassium) capable of profound neuroprotective activity.
- Thorough and extensive coverage of a complete Lyme disease detoxification program, including discussion of both liver and skin detoxification pathways. Specific detoxification therapies such as liver cleanses, bowel cleanses, the Shoemaker Neurotoxin Elimination Protocol, sauna therapy, mineral baths, mineral supplementation, milk thistle, and many others. Ideas to reduce and control herx reactions.
- Tips and clinical research from James Schaller, M.D.
- A detailed look at one method for utilizing antibiotics during a rife machine treatment campaign.
- Wide coverage of the Marshall Protocol, including an in-depth discussion of its mechanism of action in relation to Lyme disease pathology. Also, the author's personal experience with the Marshall Protocol over 3 years.
- An explanation of and new information about the Salt / Vitamin C protocol.
- Hot-off-the-press information on mangosteen fruit (not to be confused with mango) and its many benefits, including antibacterial, anti-inflammatory, and anti-cancer properties.
- New guidelines for combining all the therapies discussed in both of Rosner's books into a complete treatment plan. Brief and articulate for consideration by you and your doctor.
- Also includes updates on rife therapy, cutting-edge supplements, political challenges, an exclusive interview with Willy Burgdorfer, Ph.D. (discoverer of Lyme), and much more!

"Bryan Rosner thinks big and this new book offers big solutions."
- James Schaller, M.D.

"Another ground-breaking Lyme Disease book."
- Jeff Mittelman, moderator of the Lyme-and-rife group

"Brilliant and thorough."
- Nenah Sylver, Ph.D.

Do not miss this top Lyme disease resource. Discover new healing tools today! Bring this book to your doctor's appointment to help with forming a treatment plan.

Paperback book, 7 x 10", 367 pages, $35

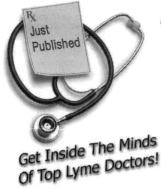

Just Published

Get Inside The Minds Of Top Lyme Doctors!

13 Lyme Doctors Share Treatment Strategies!

In this new book, not one, but thirteen Lyme-literate healthcare practitioners describe the tools they use in their practices to heal patients from chronic Lyme disease. Never before available in book format!

Insights Into Lyme Disease Treatment: 13 Lyme Literate Health Care Practitioners Share Their Healing Strategies

By Connie Strasheim
Foreword by Maureen Mcshane, M.D.

If you traveled the country for appointments with 13 Lyme-literate health care practitioners, you would discover many cutting-edge therapies used to combat chronic Lyme disease. You would also spend thousands of dollars on hotels, plane tickets, and medical appointment fees—not to mention the time it would take to embark on such a journey.

Even if you had the time and money to travel, would the physicians have enough time to answer all of your questions? Would you even know which questions to ask?

In this long-awaited book, health care journalist and Lyme patient Connie Strasheim

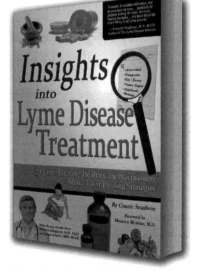

Paperback • 443 Pages • $39.95

has done all the work for you. She conducted intensive interviews with 13 of the world's most competent Lyme disease healers, asking them thoughtful, important questions, and then spent months compiling their information into 13 organized, user-friendly chapters that contain the core principles upon which they base their medical treatment of chronic Lyme disease. The practitioners' backgrounds span a variety of disciplines, including allopathic, naturopathic, complementary, chiropractic, homeopathic, and energy medicine. All aspects of treatment are covered, from anti-microbial remedies and immune system support, to hormonal restoration, detoxification, and dietary/lifestyle choices. **PHYSICIANS INTERVIEWED:**

- Steven Bock, M.D.
- Ginger Savely, DNP
- Ronald Whitmont, M.D.
- Nicola McFadzean, N.D.
- Jeffrey Morrison, M.D.
- Steven J. Harris, M.D.
- Peter J. Muran, M.D., M.B.A.

- Ingo D. E. Woitzel, M.D.
- Susan L. Marra, M.S., N.D.
- W. Lee Cowden, M.D., M.D. (H)
- Deborah Metzger, Ph.D., M.D.
- Marlene Kunold, "Heilpraktiker"
- Elizabeth Hesse-Sheehan, DC, CCN
- **Visit our website to read a <u>FREE CHAPTER</u>!**

Paperback book, 7 x 10", 443 pages, $39.95

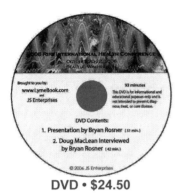

DVD • $24.50

Rife International Health Conference Feature-Length DVD (93 Minutes)

Bryan Rosner's Presentation and Interview with Doug MacLean

The Official Rife Technology Seminar Seattle, WA, USA

If you have been unable to attend the Rife International Health Conference, this DVD is your opportunity to watch two very important Lyme-related presentations from the event:

Presentation #1: Bryan Rosner's Sunday morning talk entitled *Lyme Disease: New Paradigms in Diagnosis and Treatment - the Myths, the Reality, and the Road Back to Health*. (51 minutes)

Presentation #2: Bryan Rosner's interview with Doug MacLean, in which Doug talked about his experiences with Lyme disease, including the incredible journey he undertook to invent the first modern rife machine used to fight Lyme disease. Although Doug's journey as a Lyme disease pioneer took place 20 years ago, this was the first time Doug has ever accepted an invitation to appear in public. This is the only video available where you can see Doug talk about what it was like to be the first person ever to use rife technology as a treatment for Lyme disease. Now you can see how it all began. Own this DVD and own a piece of history! (42 minutes)

Lymebook.com has secured a special licensing agreement with JS Enterprises, the Canadian producer of the Rife Conference videos, to bring this product to you at the special low price of $24.50. Total DVD viewing time: 1 hour, 33 minutes. We have DVDs in stock, shipped to you within 3 business days.

Price Comparison (should you get the DVD?)

Cost of attending the recent Rife Conference (2 people):
Hotel Room, 3 Nights = $400
Registration = $340
Food = $150
Airfare = $600
Total = $1,490

Cost of the DVD, which you can view as many times as you want, and show to family and friends:
DVD = $24.50

Bryan Rosner Presenting on Sunday Morning In Seattle

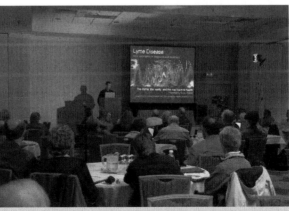

**DVD
93 Minutes
$24.50**

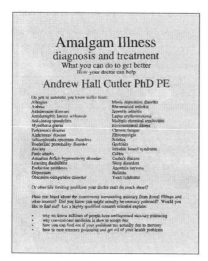

Book • $35

Amalgam Illness, Diagnosis and Treatment: What You Can Do to Get Better, How Your Doctor Can Help

By Andrew Cutler, PhD

This book was written by a chemical engineer who himself got mercury poisoning from his amalgam dental fillings. He found that there was no suitable educational material for either the patient or the physician. Knowing how much people can suffer from this condition, he wrote this book to help them get well. With a PhD in chemistry from Princeton University and extensive study in biochemistry and medicine, Andrew Cutler uses layman's terms to explain how people become mercury poisoned and what to do about it. The author's research shows that mercury poisoning can easily be cured at home with over-the-counter oral chelators – this book explains how.

In the book you will find practical guidance on how to tell if you really have chronic mercury poisoning or some other problem. Proper diagnostic procedures are provided so that sick people can decide what is wrong rather than trying random treatments. If mercury poisoning is your problem, the book tells you how to get the mercury out of your body, and how to feel good while you do that. The treatment section gives step-by-step directions to figure out exactly what mercury is doing to you and how to fix it.

"Dr. Cutler uses his background in chemistry to explain the safest approach to treat mercury poisoning. I am a physician and am personally using his protocol on myself."

- Melissa Myers, M.D.

Sections also explain how the scientific literature shows many people must be getting poisoned by their amalgam fillings, why such a regulatory blunder occurred, and how the debate between "mainstream" and "alternative" medicine makes it more difficult for you to get the medical help you need.

This down-to-earth book lets patients take care of themselves. It also lets doctors who are not familiar with chronic mercury intoxication treat it. The book is a practical guide to getting well. Sections from the book include:

- Why worry about mercury poisoning?
- What mercury does to you – symptoms, laboratory test irregularities, diagnostic checklist.
- How to treat mercury poisoning easily with oral chelators.
- Dealing with other metals including copper, arsenic, lead, cadmium.
- Dietary and supplement guidelines.
- Balancing hormones during the recovery process.
- How to feel good while you are chelating the metals out.
- How heavy metals cause infections to thrive in the body.
- Politics and mercury.

This is the world's most authoritative, accurate book on mercury poisoning.

Paperback book, 8.5 x 11", 226 pages, $35

Hair Test Interpretation: Finding Hidden Toxicities

By Andrew Cutler, PhD

Hair tests are worth doing because a surprising number of people diagnosed with incurable chronic health conditions actually turn out to have a heavy metal problem; quite often, mercury poisoning. Heavy metal problems can be corrected. Hair testing allows the underlying problem to be identified – and the chronic health condition often disappears with proper detoxification.

Hair Test Interpretation: Finding Hidden Toxicities is a practical book that explains how to interpret **Doctor's Data, Inc**. and **Great Plains Laboratory** hair tests. A step-by-step discussion is provided, with figures to illustrate the process and make it easy. The book gives examples using actual hair test results from real people.

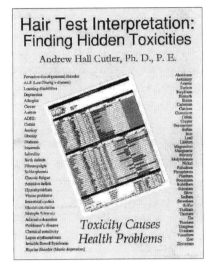

Hair Test Interpretation: Finding Hidden Toxicities

Andrew Hall Cutler, Ph. D., P. E.

Toxicity Causes Health Problems

Book • $35

One of the problems with hair testing is that both conventional and alternative health care providers do not know how to interpret these tests. Interpretation is not as simple as looking at the results and assuming that any mineral out of the reference range is a problem mineral.

Interpretation is complicated because heavy metal toxicity, especially mercury poisoning, interferes with mineral transport throughout the body. Ironically, if someone is mercury poisoned, hair test mercury is often low and other minerals may be elevated or take on unusual values. For example, mercury often causes retention of arsenic, antimony, tin, titanium, zirconium, and aluminum. An inexperienced health care provider may wrongly assume that one of these other minerals is the culprit, when in reality mercury is the true toxicity.

"This new book of Andrew's is the definitive guide in the confusing world of heavy metal poisoning diagnosis and treatment. I'm a practicing physician, 20 years now, specializing in detoxification programs for treatment of resistant conditions. It was fairly difficult to diagnose these heavy metal conditions before I met Andrew Cutler and developed a close relationship with him while reading his books. In this book I found his usual painful attention to detail gave a solid framework for understanding the complexity of mercury toxicity as well as the less common exposures. You really couldn't ask for a better reference book on a subject most researchers and physicians are still fumbling in the dark about."
- Dr. Rick Marschall

So, as you can see, getting a hair test is only the first step. The second step is figuring out what the hair test means. Andrew Cutler, PhD, is a registered professional chemical engineer with years of experience in biochemical and healthcare research. This clear and concise book makes hair test interpretation easy, so that you know which toxicities are causing your health problems.

Paperback book, 8.5 x 11", 298 pages, $35

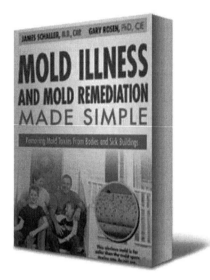
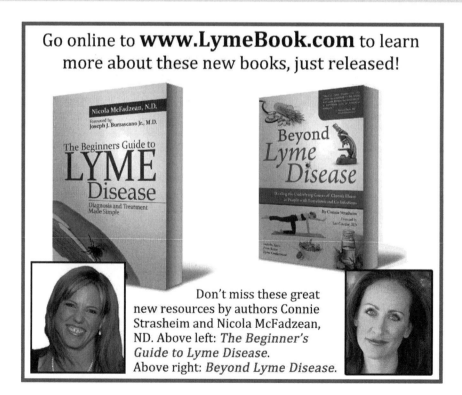

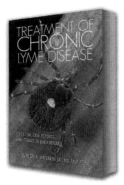
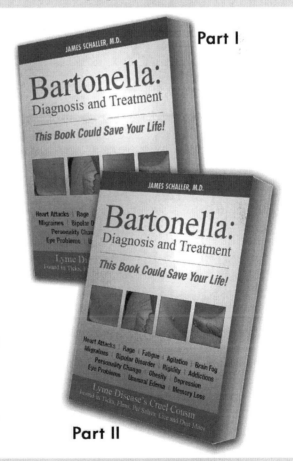

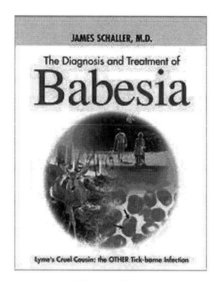

JAMES SCHALLER, M.D.

The Diagnosis and Treatment of

Babesia

Lyme's Cruel Cousin: the OTHER Tick-borne Infection

Book • $55

The Diagnosis and Treatment of Babesia: Lyme's Cruel Cousin – The Other Tick-Borne Infection

By James Schaller, M.D.

Do you or a loved one experience excess fatigue? Have you ever had unusually high fevers, chills, or sweats? You may have Babesia, a very common tick-borne infection. Babesia is often found with Lyme disease and, like all tick-borne infections, is rarely diagnosed and reported accurately.

The deer tick which carries Lyme disease and Babesia may be as small as a poppy seed and injects a painkiller, an antihistamine, and an anticoagulant to avoid detection. As a result, many people have Babesia and do not know it. Numerous forms of Babesia are carried by ticks. This book introduces patients and health care workers to the various species that infect humans and are not routinely tested for by sincere physicians.

Dr. Schaller, who practices medicine in Florida, first became interested in Babesia after one of his own children was infected with it. None of the elite pediatricians or child specialists could help. No one tested for Babesia or considered it a possible diagnosis. His child suffered from just two of these typical Babesia symptoms:

- Significant Fatigue
- Coughing
- Dizziness
- Trouble Thinking
- Fevers
- Memory Loss

- Chills
- Air Hunger
- Headache
- Sweats
- Unresponsiveness to Lyme Treatment

With 374 pages, this book is the most current and comprehensive book on Babesia in the English language. It reviews thousands of articles and presents the results of interviews with world experts on the subject. It offers you top information and broad treatment options, presented in a clear and simple manner. All treatments are explained thoroughly, including their possible side effects, drug interactions, various dosing strategies, pros/cons, and physician experiences.

"Once again Dr. Schaller has provided us with a much-needed and practical resource. This book gave me exactly what I was looking for."

- Thomas W., Patient

Finally, the book also addresses many other aspects of practical medical care often overlooked in this infection, such as treatment options for managing fatigue. Plainly stated, this book is a must-have for patients and health care providers who deal with Lyme disease and its co-infections. Dr. Schaller's many years in clinical practice give the book a practical angle that many other similar books lack. Don't miss this user-friendly resource!

Paperback book, 7 x 10", 374 pages, $55

Also available on our website as an eBook!

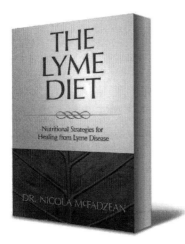

Book • $24.95

The Lyme Diet: Nutritional Strategies for Healing from Lyme Disease

By Nicola McFadzean, N.D.

We know about antibiotics and herbs. But what is the right diet for Lyme sufferers? Now you can read about the experience of Dr. Nicola McFadzean, N.D., in treating Lyme patients using proper diet.

The author is a Naturopathic Doctor and graduate of Bastyr University in Seattle, Washington. She is currently in private practice at her clinic, RestorMedicine, located in San Diego, California.

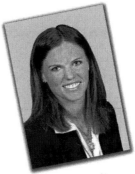

Nicola McFadzean, N.D.

This book covers numerous topics (not just diet-related):

- Reducing and controlling inflammation
- Maximizing immune function via dietary choices
- Restoring the gut & regaining healthy digestion
- Detoxification with food
- Hormone imbalances
- Biofilms
- Kefir vs. yogurt vs. probiotics
- Candida, liver support, and much more!

Paperback book, 6x9", 214 Pages, $24.95
Also available as an eBook on our website!

Cannabis for Lyme Disease & Related Conditions: Scientific Basis & Anecdotal Evidence for Medicinal Use *By Shelley White, with Foreword by Julie McIntyre, Clinical Herbalist*

Natural medicine has proven helpful for many Lyme sufferers. Unfortunately, Lyme herbalists and naturopathic doctors are relatively scarce, and treatments can be expensive. It is clear that more practical herbal treatments are in great demand. This book meets that demand, and offers an in-depth and easy-to-understand guide to walk patients through the natural treatment process. White's personal experience treating her own Lyme disease with cannabis, along with her background as a writer and researcher, inspired this book. Readers will find out about various aspects of cannabis and its medicinal uses, including its antibacterial properties, chemical constituents, strains, forms and methods of use, as well as recipes, safety, and legal considerations.

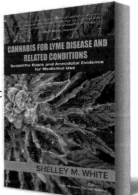

Paperback Book • $24.95

Paperback book, 6x9", 260 pages, $24.95

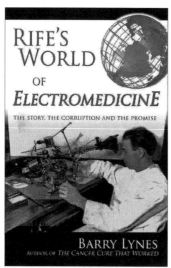

BARRY LYNES
AUTHOR OF *THE CANCER CURE THAT WORKED*

Book • $17.95

Rife's World of Electromedicine: The Story, the Corruption and the Promise

By Barry Lynes

The cause of cancer was discovered in the early 1930's. It was a virus-sized, mini-bacteria or "particle" that induced cells to become malignant and grow into tumors. The cancer microbe or particle was given the name BX by the brilliant scientist who discovered it: Royal Raymond Rife.

Laboratory verification of the cause of cancer was done hundreds of times with mice in order to be absolutely certain. Five of America's most prominent physicians helped oversee clinical trials managed by a major university's medical school.

Sixteen cancer patients were brought by ambulance twice a week to the clinical trial location in La Jolla, California. There they were treated with a revolutionary electromedicine that painlessly, non-invasively destroyed only the cancer-causing microbe or particle named BX. After just three months of this therapy, all patients were diagnosed as clinically cured. Later, the therapy was suppressed and remains so today.

In 1987, Barry Lynes wrote the classic book on Rife history (*The Cancer Cure That Worked*, see catalog page 14). *Rife's World* is the sequel.

Paperback book, 5.5 x 8.5", 90 pages, $17.95

Physicians' Desk Reference (PDR) Books (opposing page)

Most people have heard of *Physicians' Desk Reference* (PDR) books because, for over 60 years, physicians and researchers have turned to PDR for the latest word on prescription drugs.

THOMSON ™

You may not know that Thomson Healthcare, publisher of PDR, offers PDR reference books not only for drugs, but also for herbal and nutritional supplements. No available books come even close to the amount of information provided in these PDRs—*PDR for Herbal Medicines* weighs 5 lbs and has over 1300 pages, and *PDR for Nutritional Supplements* weighs over 3 lbs and has more than 800 pages.

> "I relied heavily on the PDRs during the research phase of writing my books. Without them, my projects would have greatly suffered."
>
> **- Bryan Rosner**

We carry all three PDRs. Although PDR books are typically used by physicians, we feel that these resources are also essential for people interested in or recovering from chronic disease. For the supplements, herbs, and drugs included in the books, you will find the following information: Pharmacology, description and method of action, available trade names and brands, indications and usage, research summaries, dosage options, history of use, pharmacokinetics, and much more! Worth the money for years of faithful use.

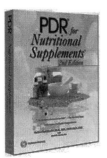

PDR for Nutritional Supplements *2nd Edition!*

This PDR focuses on the following types of supplements:

- Vitamins
- Minerals
- Amino acids
- Hormones
- Lipids
- Glyconutrients
- Probiotics
- Proteins
- Many more!

"In a part of the health field not known for its devotion to rigorous science, [this book] brings to the practitioner and the curious patient a wealth of hard facts."

- Roger Guillemin, M.D., Ph.D., Nobel Laureate in Physiology and Medicine

Book • $69.50

The book also suggests supplements that can help reduce prescription drug side effects, has full-color photographs of various popular commercial formulations (and contact information for the associated suppliers), and so much more! Become educated instead of guessing which supplements to take.

Hardcover book, 11 x 9.3", 800 pages, $69.50

PDR for Herbal Medicines *4th Edition!*

PDR for Herbal Medicines is very well organized and presents information on hundreds of common and uncommon herbs and herbal preparations. Indications and usage are examined with regard to homeopathy, Indian and Chinese medicine, and unproven (yet popular) applications.

In an area of healthcare so unstudied and vulnerable to hearsay and hype, this scientifically referenced book allows you to find out the real story behind the herbs lining the walls of your local health food store.

Use this reference before spending money on herbal products!

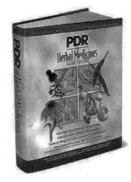

Book • $69.50

Hardcover book, 11 x 9.3", 1300 pages, $69.50

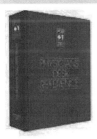

PDR for Prescription Drugs *Current Year's Edition!*

With more than 3,000 pages, this is the most comprehensive and respected book in the world on over 4,000 drugs. Drugs are indexed by both brand and generic name (in the same convenient index) and also by manufacturer and product category. This PDR provides usage information and warnings, drug interactions, plus a detailed, full-color directory with descriptions and cross references for the drugs. A new format allows dramatically improved readability and easier access to the information you need now.

Book • $99.50

Hardcover book, 12.5 x 9.5", 3533 pages, $99.50

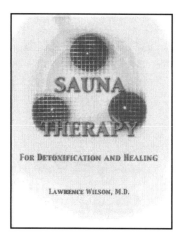

Book • $22.95

Sauna Therapy for Detoxification and Healing

By Lawrence Wilson, MD

This book provides a thorough yet articulate education on sauna therapy. It includes construction plans for a low-cost electric light sauna. The book is well referenced with an extensive bibliography.

Sauna therapy, especially with an electric light sauna, is one of the most powerful, safe and cost-effective methods of natural healing. It is especially important today due to extensive exposure to toxic metals and chemicals.

Fifteen chapters cover sauna benefits, physiological effects, protocols, cautions, healing reactions, and many other aspects of sauna therapy.

Dr. Wilson is an instructor of Biochemistry, Hair Mineral Analysis, Sauna Therapy and Jurisprudence at various colleges and universities including Yamuni Institute of the Healing Arts (Maurice, LA), University of Natural Medicine (Santa Fe, NM), Natural Healers Academy (Morristown, NJ), and Westbrook University (West Virginia). His books are used as textbooks at East-West School of Herbology and Ohio College of Natural Health. Go to www.LymeBook.com for free book excerpts!

Paperback book, 8.5 x 11", 167 pages, $22.95

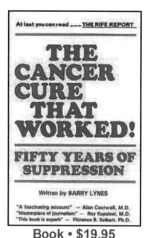

Book • $19.95

Over 50,000 Copies Sold!

The Cancer Cure That Worked: Fifty Years of Suppression

At Last You Can Read... The Rife Report

By Barry Lynes

Investigative journalism at its best. Barry Lynes takes readers on an exciting journey into the life work of Royal Rife. **We are now the official publisher of this book. Call or visit us online for wholesale terms.**

"A fascinating account..." **-Alan Cantwell, MD**

"This book is superb." **-Florence B. Seibert, PhD**

"Barry Lynes is one of the greatest health reporters in our country. With the assistance of John Crane, longtime friend and associate of Roy Rife, Barry has produced a masterpiece..." **-Roy Kupsinel, M.D., editor of *Health Consciousness Journal***

Paperback book, 5 x 8", 169 pages, $19.95

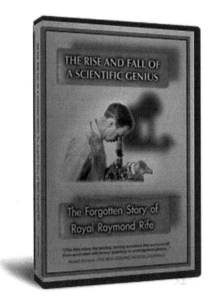

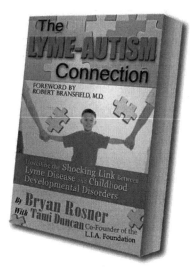

Book • $25.95

The Lyme-Autism Connection: Unveiling the Shocking Link Between Lyme Disease and Childhood Developmental Disorders

By Bryan Rosner & Tami Duncan

Did you know that Lyme disease may contribute to the onset of autism?

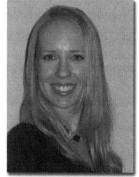

This book is an investigative report written by Bryan Rosner and Tami Duncan. Duncan is the co-founder of the *Lyme Induced Autism (LIA) Foundation*, and her son has an autism diagnosis.

Tami Duncan, Co-Founder of the Lyme Induced Autism (LIA) Foundation

Awareness of the Lyme-autism connection is spreading rapidly, among both parents and practitioners. *Medical Hypothesis*, a scientific, peer-reviewed journal published by Elsevier, recently released an influential study entitled *The Association Between Tick-Borne Infections, Lyme Borreliosis and Autism Spectrum Disorders*. Here is an excerpt from the study:

> "Chronic infectious diseases, including tick-borne infections such as Borrelia burgdorferi, may have direct effects, promote other infections, and create a weakened, sensitized and immunologically vulnerable state during fetal development and infancy, leading to increased vulnerability for developing autism spectrum disorders. An association between Lyme disease and other tick-borne infections and autistic symptoms has been noted by numerous clinicians and parents."

—Medical Hypothesis Journal.
Article Authors: Robert C. Bransfield, M.D., Jeffrey S. Wulfman, M.D., William T. Harvey, M.D., Anju I. Usman, M.D.

Nationwide, 1 out of 150 children are diagnosed with Autism Spectrum Disorder (ASD), and the LIA Foundation has discovered that many of these children test positive for Lyme disease/Borrelia related complex—yet most children in this scenario never receive appropriate medical attention. This book answers many difficult questions: How can infants contract Lyme disease if autism begins before birth, precluding the opportunity for a tick bite? Is there a statistical correlation between the incidences of Lyme disease and autism worldwide? Do autistic children respond to Lyme disease treatment? What does the medical community say about this connection? Do the mothers of affected children exhibit symptoms? **Find out in this book.**

Paperback book, 6x9", 287 pages, $25.95

Dietrich Klinghardt, M.D., Ph.D. "Fundamental Teachings" 5-DVD Set

Includes Disc Exclusively For Lyme Disease!

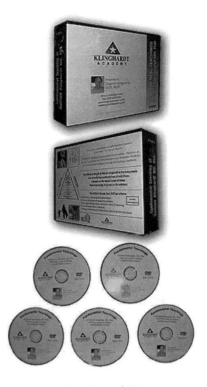

Dietrich Klinghardt, M.D., Ph.D. is a legendary healer known for discovering and refining many of the cutting-edge treatment protocols used for a variety of chronic health problems including Lyme disease, autism and mercury poisoning.

Now you can find out all about this doctor's treatment methods from the privacy of your own home! This 5-DVD set includes the following DVDs:

- **DISC 1**: The Five Levels of Healing and the Seven Factors
- **DISC 2**: Autonomic Response Testing and Demonstration
- **DISC 3**: Heavy Metal Toxicity and Neurotoxin Elimination / Electrosmog
- **DISC 4:** Lyme disease and Chronic Illness
- **DISC 5**: Psycho-Emotional Issues in Chronic Illness & Addressing Underlying Causes

5-DVD Set • $125

Dr. Dietrich Klinghardt is one of the most important contributors to modern integrative treatment for Lyme disease and related medical conditions. This comprehensive DVD set is a must-have addition to your educational library.

5-DVD Set, $125

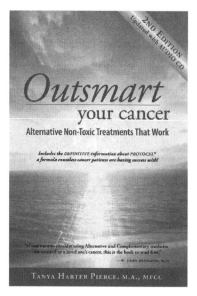

Book and Audio CD • $26.95

<u>2nd Edition!</u> **Outsmart Your Cancer: Alternative Non-Toxic Treatments That Work   By Tanya Harter Pierce**

Why BLUDGEON cancer to death with common conventional treatments that can be toxic and harmful to your entire body?

When you OUTSMART your cancer, only the cancer cells die — NOT your healthy cells! *OUTSMART YOUR CANCER: Alternative Non-Toxic Treatments That Work* is an easy guide to successful non-toxic treatments for cancer that you can obtain right now! In it, you will read real-life stories of people who have completely recovered from their advanced or late-stage lung cancer, breast cancer, prostate cancer, kidney cancer, brain cancer, childhood leukemia, and other types of cancer using effective non-toxic approaches.

Plus, *OUTSMART YOUR CANCER* is one of the few books in print today that gives a complete description of the amazing formula called "Protocel," which has produced incredible cancer recoveries over the past 20 years. **A supporting audio CD is included with this book**.

Paperback book, 6 x 9", 437 pages, with audio CD, $26.95

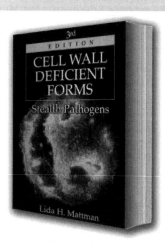

Hardcover Book • $169.95

Cell Wall Deficient Forms: Stealth Pathogens

By Lida Mattman, Ph.D.

This is one of the most influential infectious disease textbook of the century. Dr. Mattman, who earned a Ph.D. in immunology from Yale University, describes her discovery that a certain type of pathogen lacking a cell wall is the root cause of many of today's "incurable" and mysterious chronic diseases. Dr. Mattman's research is the foundation of our current understanding of Lyme disease, and her work led to many of the Lyme protocols used today (such as the Marshall Protocol, as well as modern LLMD antibiotic treatment strategy). Color illustrations and meticulously referenced breakthrough principles cover the pages of this book. A must have for all serious students of chronic, elusive infectious disease.

Hardcover book, 7.5 x 10.5", 416 pages, $169.95

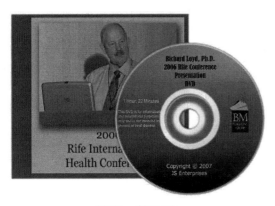

DVD • $24.50

Richard Loyd, Ph.D., presents at the Rife International Health Conference in Seattle

Watch this DVD to gain a better understanding of the technical details of rife technology.

Dr. Loyd, who earned a Ph.D. in nutrition, has researched and experimented with numerous electrotherapeutic devices, including the Rife/Bare unit, various EMEM machines, F-Scan, BioRay, magnetic pulsers, Doug Machine, and more. Dr. Loyd also has a wealth of knowledge in the use of herbs and supplements to support Rife electromagnetics.

By watching this DVD, you will discover the nuts and bolts of some very important, yet little known, principles of rife machine operation, including:

- Gating, sweeping, session time
- Square vs. sine wave
- DC vs. AC frequencies
- Duty cycle
- Octaves and scalar octaves

- Voltage variations and radio frequencies
- Explanation of the spark gap
- Contact vs. radiant mode
- Stainless vs. copper contacts
- A unique look at various frequency devices

DVD, 57 minutes, $24.50

Under Our Skin: Lyme Disease Documentary Film

A gripping tale of microbes, medicine & money, UNDER OUR SKIN exposes the hidden story of Lyme disease, one of the most serious and controversial epidemics of our time. Each year, thousands go undiagnosed or misdiagnosed, often told that their symptoms are all in their head. Following the stories of patients and physicians fighting for their lives and livelihoods, the film brings into focus a haunting picture of the health care system and a medical establishment all too willing to put profits ahead of patients.

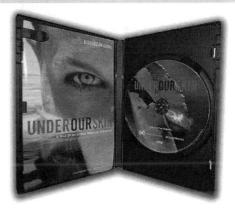

DVD • $34.95

Bonus Features: 32-page discussion guidebook, one hour of bonus footage, director's commentary, and much more! FOR HOME USE ONLY

DVD with bonus features, 104 minutes, $34.95 *MUST SEE!*

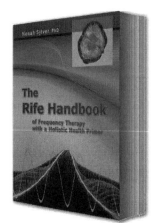

INDEX

5-HTP, 102–4, 156, 222, 227–28, 230, 242

A

A-BAB, 225
A-BART, 225
Acetyladehydes, 97–98, 140
Acetylcholine, 23, 73, 104–6, 110, 116, 241
Acetyl-L-carnitine, 106, 114–16, 121, 123,
    222, 227, 284, 291–92
Adderall, 72
Addiction, 70, 72, 104, 228
ADHD (attention deficit hyperactivity disor-
    ders), 22, 72, 118, 210
Adrenals, 148, 155–56, 161, 193, 199–200,
    276
Aerobic exercise, 159–62, 283
Alcohol, 69, 71, 97, 115, 140, 146–47,
    154–55, 254
A-L Complex, 224
Alinia, 50, 57
Alkaloids, 81, 85, 283
Allergies, 58, 98, 134–36, 252, 254
Allicin, 79
Allimax, 79
Aloe vera Powder, 228
Alpha-linolenic acid, 88, 117
Alpha-lipoic acid, 57, 116–17, 124, 196, 222,
    289, 292
Aluminum, 88, 195, 303
Alzheimer's disease, 15–16, 24, 73, 93, 104,
    107, 110, 113, 116, 118–19, 124, 252,
    283, 286–87, 290
Amalgam dental fillings, 302
Ambient air, 188
Ammonia, 21–22, 98–99, 235–37, 243
Amoxicillin, 49, 52, 54–55
Amygdala, 178, 255
Anaplasma, 28–29, 56, 289
Andrographis, 79–81, 85, 222, 224
Anise, 97, 226
Annual Rife International Health Conference,
    298, 311
Anorexia, 246, 272
Anticoagulant, 20, 306
Anticonvulsant, 99, 285
Antihistamines, 70, 157, 306
Antipsychotics, 28, 65, 67
Anti-thyroglobulin, 202
Apathy, 73, 104

Arsenic, 116, 206, 302–3
Artemisinin, 83–85, 222, 224, 229
Arthritis, 88–89, 170
Artificial sweeteners, 60
Aspartame, 141–42
Asthma, 71, 88
Astragalus, 224–25
Atovaquone, 50, 57–58, 291
Autism, 4, 22–23, 60, 66, 188, 213, 239, 242,
    312–13
Autoimmune disease, 61, 87, 252
Avocados, 143–44
Axons, 17, 181, 188
Azithromycin, 49, 53, 55–56

B

Bactrim, 58
Bastyr University, 295, 307
Bb Tox, 21, 25, 282
Beam Ray machine, 311
Bell's Palsy, 89, 273
Benadryl, 70–71
Benzathine, 49
Benzodiazepines, 28, 65, 70–72, 104, 242
Berenbaum, Sandy, 40, 217, 245, 249, 267,
    280
Beta-blockers, 70–71
BetterHealthGuy.com, 239
Biaxin, 49
Bicillin L-A, 49, 51–54
Bilberry, 224
Bile ducts, 150
Biofilm, 54–55, 91, 307
Biotoxins, 22, 236
Bipolar disorder, 4, 64–66, 94, 110–11, 118,
    215–16, 280, 285
Black mold, 203
Black pepper, 126
Black tea extract, 226
Black walnut, 224
Blueberries, 136, 141
Bluetooth devices, 155, 205
Blumea balsamifera, 225
Body brushing, 243
Boswellia, 88–89, 92, 222, 226, 228, 286, 292
Bottled water, 206
Brain edema, 85, 89–90, 288
Brain stem, 154, 251
Bransfield, Robert C., 1–2, 24, 39, 177–78,
    251, 255–56, 269, 282, 312

Printed in Great Britain
by Amazon